THE
ADVENTUROUS
EATERS CLUB

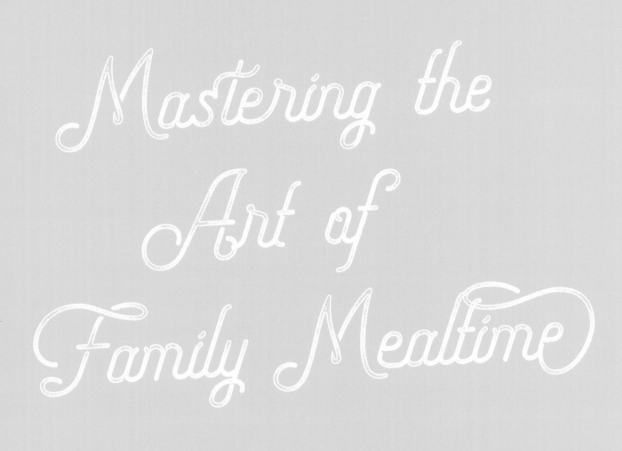

Mastering the
Art of
Family Mealtime

THE
ADVENTUROUS
EATERS CLUB

Misha and Vicki Collins

Photography by Michèle M. Waite

HarperOne
An Imprint of HarperCollinsPublishers

HarperOne

HarperCollins books may be purchased for educational, business, or sales promotional use. For information, please email the Special Markets Department at SPsales@harpercollins.com.

FIRST EDITION

Designed by Janet Evans-Scanlon

Photography by Michèle M. Waite

Library of Congress Cataloging-in-Publication Data

Names: Collins, Misha, author. | Collins, Vicki, author.
Title: The adventurous eaters club : mastering the art of family mealtime / Misha and Vicki Collins.
Description: San Francisco, CA : HarperOne, an imprint of HarperCollinsPublishers, 2019. | Includes bibliographical references.
Identifiers: LCCN 2019030694 (print) | LCCN 2019030695 (ebook) | ISBN 9780062876881 (hardcover) | ISBN 9780062876898 (ebook)
Subjects: LCSH: Cooking.
Classification: LCC TX714 .C614 2019 (print) | LCC TX714 (ebook) | DDC 641.5—dc23
LC record available at https://lccn.loc.gov/2019030694
LC ebook record available at https://lccn.loc.gov/2019030695

19 20 21 22 23   LSC   10 9 8 7 6 5 4 3 2 1

To West and Maison,
and all the other young,
budding adventurous eaters
in the world

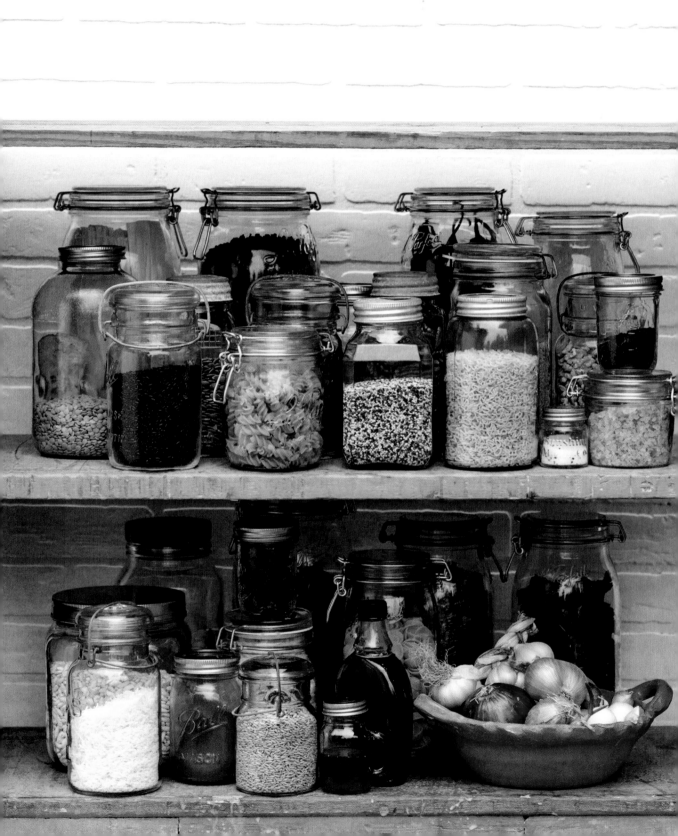

CONTENTS

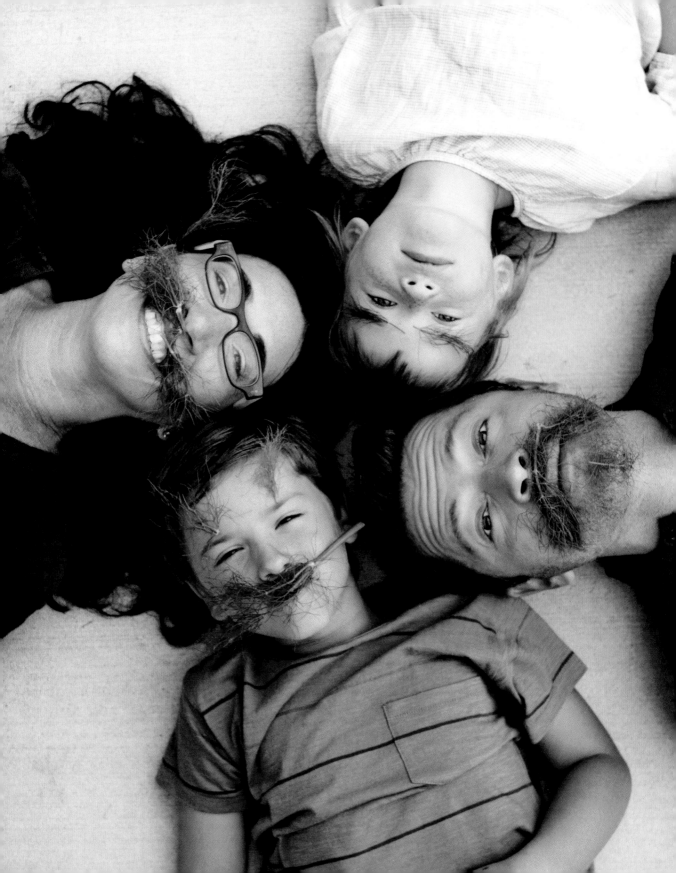

MISHA'S INTRODUCTION

I was raised poor. My mom bought groceries with food stamps, and we'd get a hot meal and a bag of dry goods every Wednesday at our local soup kitchen. Even though fancy foods like pork chops were birthday-only events, food was sacred in my family. My mom would always find a way to cook dinner for my brother and me, even when we lived in a cramped office space (without a kitchen) or a tent in the woods. Sometimes we ate over a campfire, but we sat and ate together every night. Meals were a way we conveyed love.

My mother also helped get me interested in eating a variety of foods by letting me "help" and experiment with cooking from a very young age. And it worked. I loved cooking, and I ate pretty much everything except chicken liver as a kid. I created my own recipe for apple pastries when I was seven. They were harder than oak (and about as tasty), but my mother told me they were the best she ever had.

When my wife, Vicki, and I had kids of our own, I imagined we would do some of the same things. We would feed our kids home-cooked meals; we'd let them be part of the cooking process; we'd show love with food. But then the reality of toddlers and jobs and sleeplessness set in, and we found ourselves serving our kids a lot of squeezable fruit packs and barking at them to keep away while we rushed to reheat their noodles. Feeding the kids started to feel like a race against hunger tantrums and just another chore for us to slog through. And, depressingly, the kids seemed to only have eyes for fruit chews and pasta. When we were traveling, and we traveled often, we would pick grilled cheese off the children's menu at the airport and cross our fingers that they would eat.

Then one day, something miraculous happened. We discovered that grocery shopping with the stroller was actually easier than lugging grocery bags by hand on the walk home. One day I brought our stroller to the grocery store along with our son, West, who was not yet three. When we got back to the apartment, I started unpacking in the kitchen and found some unexpected surprises. Without my noticing, West had loaded a bag of pork rinds, a bottle of fish sauce, a few Jerusalem artichokes, some canned ham, and a package of candy corn into the shopping cart. Holding up a Jerusalem artichoke, I said, "Westy, I don't even know how to cook these." Without missing a beat, he said, "I'll show you." And he did. He smashed them with a rolling pin, then instructed me to turn on the stove and we fried them until they smoked. Then he slathered peanut butter on them. It was, all in all, hilarious. And, oddly, West devoured them (I admit they were kind of tasty).

That day marked a reset for our family. We started letting West and his younger sister, Maison, occasionally lead in the kitchen. They would call us their "soo seffs" (sous chefs), and we noticed that when they participated in meal preparation, they would be proud and they would be curious and they would try new foods. Their palates started to expand beyond pasta and saltines. They started coveting salad. Devouring brussels sprouts and salmon skins. It felt like a breakthrough. Remarkably, it also felt fun. Cooking and mealtime were becoming something we all looked forward to. Something that brought us together and made us all laugh.

If I'm a nerd, which I am, my wife, Vicki, is nerd squared. When I became a TV actor, she got a PhD. And when Vicki gets curious about something, she dives deep. So when we started having mealtime breakthroughs with our kids, she rolled up her sleeves and read every study she could find on kids and food. We discovered that many of the "truths" that modern Americans take for granted—for example, that kids are only capable of enjoying bland, beige foods—are in fact *not true*. They eat bland, beige foods because that's what American children's menus have trained them to eat. Other places in the world *don't have children's menus*, and the kids eat what grown-ups eat. Other countries don't have fruit packs, and the kids eat . . . wait for it . . . fruit! By giving in to the ubiquitous American kids' menu, we are teaching our children to eat only familiar, homogenous processed foods. In doing so, we're not only instilling restrictive, unhealthy eating habits, we're also squelching their opportunity to discover the joyous adventure that food can be.

But there's good news. With a little patience and attention, these habits can be unlearned. Junky foods and rushed meals can become the exception, and exceptional meals that bring the family together and build love and fun can become the rule. We sincerely hope that this book will help your family move toward happy, adventurous eating, just as the happy accident of pork rinds and Jerusalem artichokes landing in our grocery bag set our family on a new course. As Maison says, "Bond appletreet!"

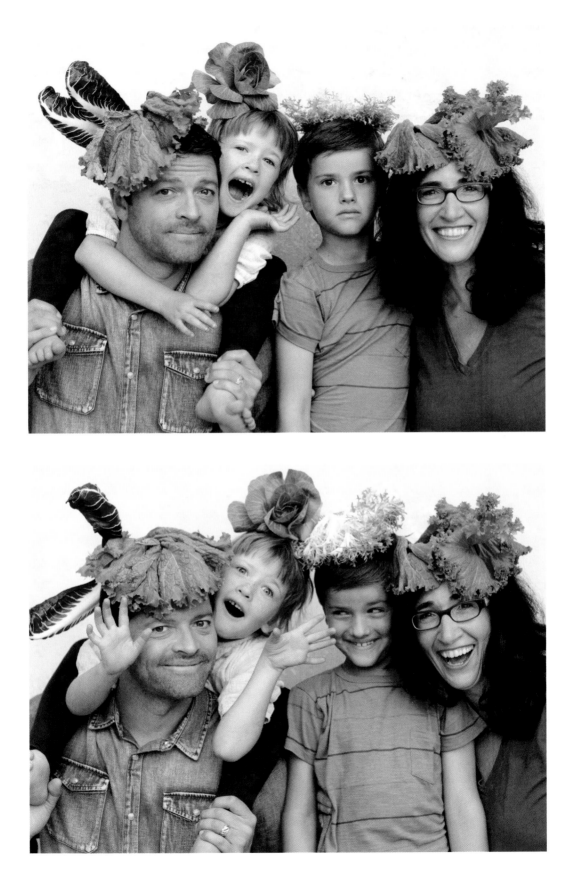

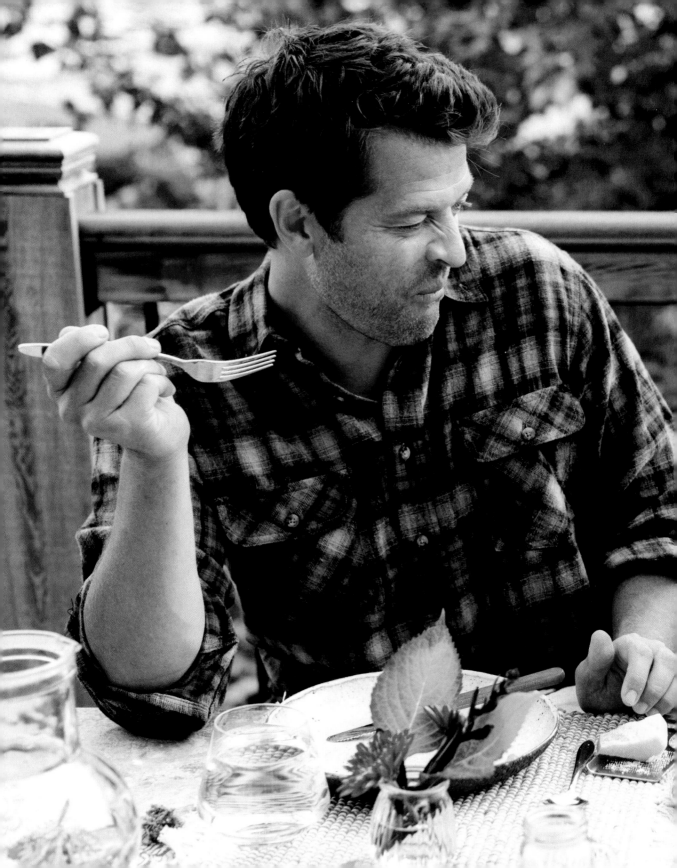

PART I

JOIN THE CLUB

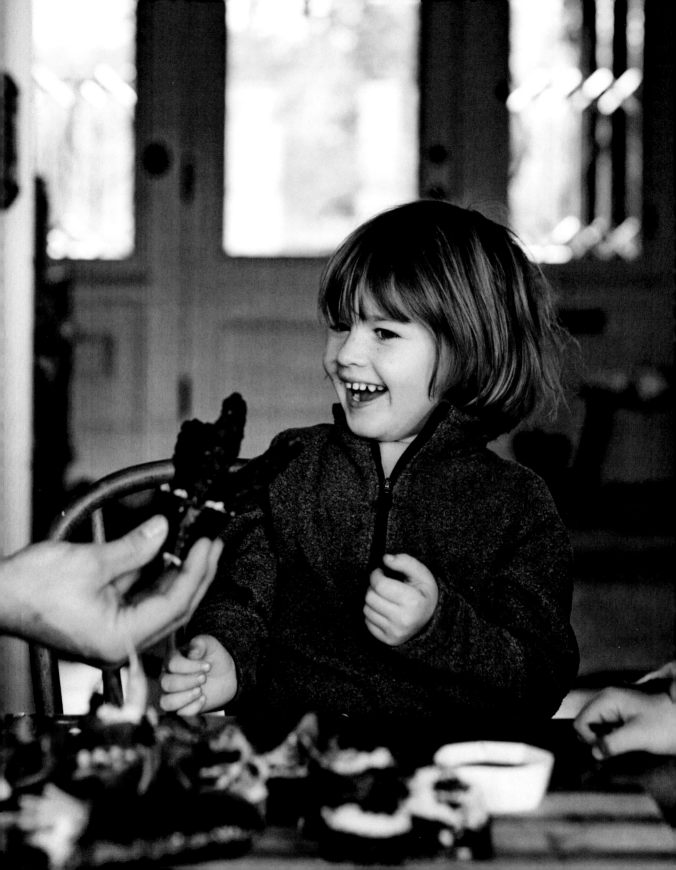

CHAPTER 1

THERE'S ANOTHER WAY TO EAT WITH KIDS

DURING OUR FIRST few years of parenting, we found mealtime downright stressful. We knew that human children needed to eat every day, but like many parents, we felt overworked, exhausted, rushed, and generally too busy to think, let alone cook. We'd sit down for dinner with our toddler son and brace ourselves. He'd hurl broccoli at us, laugh maniacally, then abruptly leave the table without consuming a single calorie. When he'd inevitably get "hangry" an hour or two later, he'd turn into a monster, clobbering innocent kids on the monkey bars. For the good of everyone at the playground, we really needed him to *eat*.

Like many well-meaning parents in the US, we fell into a pattern of shoving snacks into our child's mouth all day long. We'd leave the house armed with pockets full of crackers and fruit snacks and he'd nibble his way through the day. Of course, when mealtime rolled around, he wouldn't be hungry and he wouldn't eat dinner. We couldn't connect the dots. We thought: He just doesn't like real food. And so the cycle continued.

Not only were we perennially on edge about our son's food consumption, we also felt guilty for feeding him so many processed snacks. We really wanted him to eat fresh food. We were envious of foodie homesteader parents who grew their own cucumbers and made chia-packed muffins from scratch and had children who ate them. We felt like slackers, but we couldn't figure out how to get our kid to eat healthy meals. Besides, we didn't have time to cook anyway, so what was the point? It was all too overwhelming, and when his baby sister was born, it only felt harder.

In the midst of these mealtime battles, it feels like a no-brainer to decide that a plate of french fries smothered in ketchup, while not ideal, must be better than no food at all. Calories consumed = a win.

But when we approached food this way, we knew we were missing something. By taking processed-food shortcuts with our kids and serving them an endless rotation of beige foods, we're not only setting them up for a lifetime of health problems and boring food, we're also setting them up to miss out on the joy and adventure that food can be.

Food can connect us not only to our own bodies—to our place on earth, to the seasons—but also to each other, to our shared past, to our heritage, to other cultures. Before having kids, as a couple, we prided ourselves on our adventurousness, rebelliousness, and curiosity: we considered these qualities fundamental to who we were in the world. Some of our favorite pre-kid memories come from exploring the world together—particularly, breaking bread with new friends in unfamiliar places (we'll never forget drinking warm yak-butter tea on the Tibetan Plateau or feasting on homemade dal with our host family in Mumbai). But when we had kids, we found ourselves too exhausted to be those people anymore and too tired to teach our kids those values. The way we fed our kids (hurriedly and unimaginatively) was out of line with the adventurous selves that got tucked away as we navigated diapers, naps, and bibs. We knew we had to change *something* (besides diapers).

The Kids' Menu Takes a Toll on Health

As kids in the US have become more reliant on a narrow range of "kids' foods," their fruit and vegetable consumption has sharply declined. From 2007 to 2010, 93 percent of US children did not meet current recommendations for vegetable intake. A 2001 study of kids' menus at the top five hundred American chain restaurants found that of nearly two thousand menu options, 710 contained french fries. For the main course, more than half the entrées were fried; most of the rest were burgers or pasta. The closest thing to a vegetable on kids' menus is the carrot stick.

We all know processed food isn't good for us, but what exactly is it? Processed foods exist on a spectrum. Technically, any food that's been altered or prepared in advance for convenience is considered a processed food. Frozen veggies and roasted nuts are all processed foods—but they still live in the neighborhood of real food. It's the heavily processed foods that nutritionists find troubling. Highly processed foods include those with ingredients added for flavor and texture (including cake mix, croissants in tubes, deli meats, protein bars, packaged baked goods, and most bread) and premade meals like frozen pizza and microwaveable dinners.

These foods are laboratory-designed to be tasty, and they make parents' lives more convenient.

But they've also taken a toll on kids' health. In 2016, 18.5 percent of kids in the US were obese, according to the Centers for Disease Control and Prevention. Added sugars and solid fats constitute 40 percent of the calories eaten daily by children in the US, according to a 2018 study published in the *Journal of the American Dietetic Association.* Many children suffer from conditions such as acid reflux, low energy, and chronic constipation—all of which are typical side effects from consuming too much processed food.

The standard American kids' diet consists primarily of processed foods such as pizza, burgers, french fries, and bread, all of which are low in fiber, since processing strips food of fiber. Fiber is essential for many reasons. For one thing, it slows down carb absorption, which helps us feel satisfied, helps our bodies feel full, and signals us to stop eating. (Translation: we're more likely to overeat when eating processed foods.) Fiber also keeps our digestive systems on track, and without enough of it, our systems get thrown off and plugged up. Given the volume of processed foods consumed, it's not surprising that there are more than 2.5 million doctor visits per year in the US initiated by people who complain of constipation.

The Rise of the Chicken Finger

If the modern kids' menu isn't healthy, how did it become the cornerstone of children's diets in the US? How did this garbage become so normalized for kids? How did we get here?

A combination of factors contributed to the rise of the kids' menu—including savvy food-company marketing, busy family life, convenience-driven culture, and misguided assumptions about food preferences. Food-industry marketing teams found they could sell more packaged foods by creating separate meals specifically designed for kids. Big food companies spend a fortune marketing processed kids' meals to families. If we want our kids to eat whole and diverse foods, we're fighting an uphill battle against cultural norms and multibillion-dollar advertising campaigns.

Many parents (at least in the US) are convinced that kids can only eat ketchup-covered bland foods and that expecting anything more is totally unreasonable, possibly even negligent. Once we start believing that's all children will eat, we keep serving it, and soon children expect these familiar beige options at every meal. Many parents are brainwashed to believe that children are born with a deep resistance to vegetables. We've come to think that the only way a kid will eat a green vegetable is if we cajole, bribe, or sneak it into a Pop-Tart. But this is not true, and it's just not how families eat in the rest of the world.

> *Modern meals marketed to children send the message that if you are a kid, you cannot be expected to find enjoyment in anything so boring as real, whole food. The kids' foods in supermarkets, laced with sugar and adorned with happy cartoons, teach children that what they eat must be a form of entertainment, portable packages of fun. . . . The entire thrust of postwar commercial children's food was to make it seem "normal" for a child never to eat anything nutritious.*
>
> —BEE WILSON,
> *First Bite: How We Learn to Eat*

Kids Eat What They're Taught to Eat

This may come as a shock, but kids don't come out of the womb genetically predisposed to eat macaroni coated in slippery neon-orange pseudo–cheese sauce. Cultures around the world demonstrate that children can be taught to eat a wide range of foods.

In Korea, parents keep feeding their kids kimchi until they learn to love it—even if the kids spit it out during their first attempts. Parents in Mexico feed their babies fruit seasoned with chili powder to teach them to eat spice from an early age. While most American kids wouldn't dream of eating calamari or stinky blue cheese, in France, teachers and parents begin "taste training" at a young age, and kids learn to joyfully eat everything from fondue to liver pâté. French parents expect their kids to eat the same foods the adults eat.

"At the core of the French approach is the belief that you teach kids to eat just as you can teach them to read," says Karen Le Billon, author of *French Kids Eat Everything*. French parents consider knowing how to enjoy food a critical life skill, and they employ various strategies to "gently pry open the natural fussiness that most small children exhibit to some degree, opening their little minds and palates to a world of flavor," according to Le Billon.

Simply put, food preferences are *learned*. Kids may have varying sensitivity levels, but studies show that young children have a remarkable ability to learn to accept *and enjoy* a wide range of foods. While Japanese toddlers nibble on fermented soybean paste and kids in Burkina Faso navigate millet-seed porridge, American children are scarfing breaded chicken strips and sugar-crusted Frosted Flakes. All food is kids' food. It's perfectly possible not only to learn to *eat* all kinds of foods (including vegetables) but also to learn to *love* them. So we invite you to dump the bogus cultural assumptions about what kids eat and start fresh, just like our family did.

Eat the Damn Spinach or Else! Threats, Cajoling, and Other Strategies That Don't Work

Many of us are all too familiar with the tears and tantrums that can come from trying to force a child to eat. How many of us have threatened to put the kibosh on screen time when kids refuse their veggies . . . or bribed a kid to consume a single string bean by offering an Oreo as a reward? Coaxing, cajoling, threatening, and negotiating have become the norm at family dinner tables around the country. Welcome to the club.

In our house, we have tried pretty much every single one of these common (albeit entirely ineffective) strategies more often than we care to admit. These approaches did exactly nothing to inspire our kids to eat. Instead, our little angels just clenched their teeth.

When food becomes a battleground, it's nerve-wracking for everyone, including parents. When we started researching studies on kids and food, we found that many of our go-to tactics were, in fact, reinforcing and perpetuating this limited kids'-food diet, amplifying food-related anxiety, and setting our kids up for a long-term, messed-up relationship with food.

The American Academy of Pediatrics' nutrition guide sums it up: "It's a mistake to encourage, persuade, or bribe a child to eat. Research has shown that such efforts have the opposite effect from what's intended, and the child may actually end up eating less than if left alone." In fact, studies show that parental attempts to coerce kids into eating a particular food makes that food *less* appealing to them.

The equation is counterintuitive but simple: the more we pressure, the less kids feel like eating. I know what you're thinking: "This is totally unfair! Kids are so small and helpless: they should be much easier to control and manipulate!" We get it. We're right there with you.

Back in the 1980s, when we were kids, many parents used the classic pressure strategy known as the "clean plate club" to get kids to eat. This tactic effectively trains kids to use the visual cue of the empty plate instead of their own internal feelings of hunger and fullness to

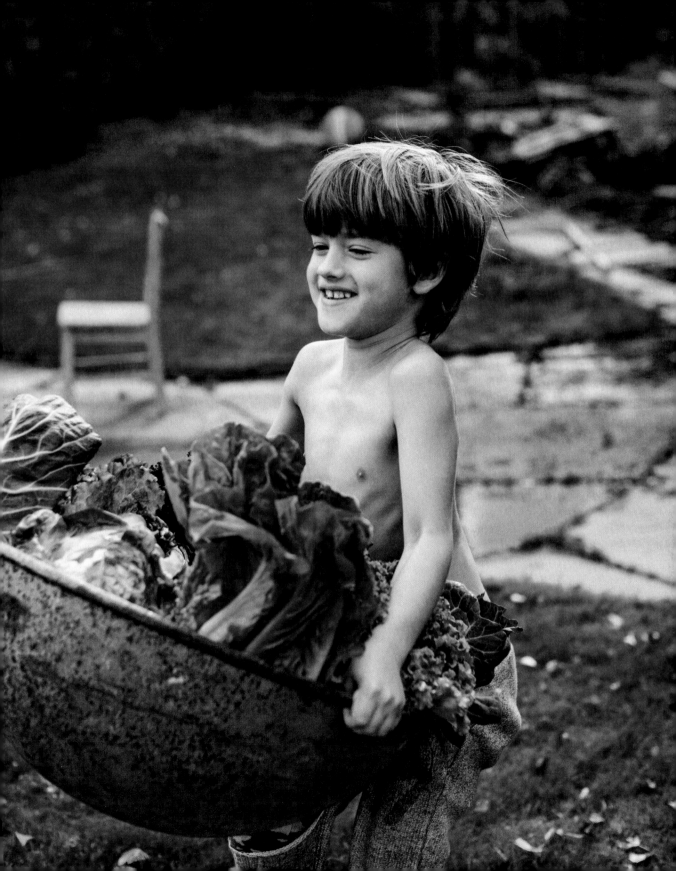

WHAT KIND OF PARENT ARE YOU?

We've tried every imaginable pitch to persuade our kids to eat. Pressure takes many forms including cheering, threatening, and bribing. Typically, American parents assume one or more of the following roles to influence their kids' eating habits:

The Dictator
You have to eat this. You won't leave the table until you eat it.

The Beggar
Pretty please, just try it.

The Compromiser
Just have two bites, then you can be done.

The Negotiator
Eat your salad, then you can have a cookie.

The Sneak
I swear, this brownie has no vegetables hidden in it.

The Cheerleader
I'm so proud of you for eating this!

The Guilt-Tripper
I worked on this meal for hours. You can at least try it!

The Salesperson
It's so yummy, you'll *love* it.

The Health Adviser
Don't you want to be big and strong? Then eat the salad.

The Minimizer
They're just potatoes! Try them!

tell them when it's time to stop eating. In the long term, the clean-plate paradigm contributes to obesity and fosters an unhealthy relationship with food. Ultimately, we want children to be attuned to their own internal cues ("Am I still hungry?" "Am I satisfied?") rather than looking to arbitrary external indicators like a clean plate or the smile of an approving dad.

Experts also advise against bribing kids to eat. Promising a sweet reward in exchange for consuming a certain quantity of food seems like a no-brainer—and yet this approach can go sideways fast. Next thing you know, your kid expects ice cream as a reward for consuming a plate of french fries. This strategy teaches kids to eat for external validation rather than paying attention to their own bodies' needs.

Studies show that using junk food as a reward for good behavior ("If you finish your homework, you can have some jelly beans") has the unintended consequence of intensifying kids' preferences for those less healthful "reward" foods. It is our ethical obligation to confess that, although we are aware that candy bribes are not considered good parenting, we've resorted to them on more than one occasion.

When it comes down to it, many parents would rather let kids eat whatever they want rather than continue the conflict.

This mind-set leads to what experts call permissive feeding. "Permissive Feeding is particularly problematic because it doesn't set up boundaries for children allowing them to strengthen their self-control. . . . If they want a food, they can have it anytime. If they are just slightly hungry, they get food the instant they say so," according to Maryann Jacobsen, author of *How to Raise a Mindful Eater*. Since this type of feeding allows children to be in charge of the menu, it usually results in a steady rotation of familiar processed kids' foods.

The Dream of Real Food

Most of us know we should be feeding our kids more fruits and vegetables. Most of us also know that it's not easy to change a family's eating habits.

When our kids were little, meals were *beyond* stressful. Our wish list was simple. We wanted our kids to eat mostly real food, to approach new food with an open sense of curiosity, and to enjoy it. Ideally, we want them to grow up to eat balanced meals without feeling guilty or obsessing about always eating healthy. It'd be dreamy if they feel internally motivated to choose healthful foods, eat regularly, and use internal cues of hunger and fullness to guide their eating. We also wanted food to be a source of connection, even pleasure, in our family. That all sounded right . . . but it seemed impossible to achieve.

We started to wonder if there was another way. Could family meals become a peaceful (or possibly even fun) experience that connected us? We started to ask ourselves: How can we buck the insidious kids'-menu brainwashing? How can we flip the script? Can we send the chicken finger to the guillotine *and* have some fun along the way?

Welcome to Adventure-Style Cooking

This book *isn't* about persuading kids to eat something they don't want to eat—it's about welcoming children into the kitchen and inviting them to become adventurous cooks and lifelong food lovers. Our mission is to inspire families to cook (and eat) together in joyous, simple, and all-embracing ways.

It wasn't easy for our family to find its path to happy, healthful family meals. We read everything we could find related to kids and food. We consulted experts of various stripes from nutritionists to child psychologists to psychics. We found that there's remarkable consensus among experts on strategies for developing health and harmony around food. Drawing on nutrition studies, child development research, interviews with teachers, advice from families who happily eat real food together, as well as literature written by pediatricians, occupational therapists, and psychologists, we've culled and distilled the morsels we've found most useful for reinventing our own family's relationship with food. Over time, we implemented many of these best practices.

This book also draws on many not-at-all-scientific experiments we've conducted in our own kitchen laboratory. When food felt like a struggle in our family, we decided to lean in to what we love best—adventure. We began to experiment: we set our two-year-old son free in a supermarket. (Experts advise against this and pretty much anyone who's ever met a toddler knows this is a truly terrible idea.) Toddler West could choose any groceries he wanted and use them to prepare dinner with a parent sous chef. One evening our son served us a warm mélange of marshmallows, carrots, and canned ham. He's still waiting for his well-deserved Michelin star.

Even though our family's homegrown adventure cooking methods are not 100 percent effective, we've found that the dynamics around food in our family are changing for the better. Rather than girding for a fight at dinner, we enjoy meals together. We found that encouraging our kids to explore in the kitchen has led to

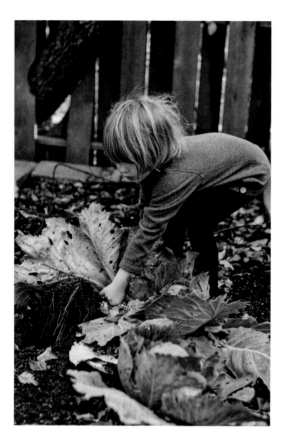

coming children into the kitchen, saying "yes, *and*" to their culinary curiosities, and exploring food together. We see family cooking as a messy, fun adventure. Things don't have to be perfect, and there's no right way.

What if your kid suggests making the world's biggest salad in the bathtub? Go for it. What about a banana pizza? Absolutely. Our family's cooking philosophy is this: let your kids add cinnamon to the peas if they want to. And don't freak out when they add too much or too little of something. Pancakes will sometimes come out simultaneously burned and undercooked. Milk will undoubtedly be spilled. Encourage your kids to bring their unique personalities and vision into cooking without worrying about doing it "right." If that means a few eggshells in the batter, so be it. If your little one isn't ready to try a certain ingredient or has ideas for fine-tuning a recipe, we encourage you to go ahead and stray from the recipe.

Many of the recipes in this book came from improvising in the kitchen with our kids—and following their lead. After all, preparing food can be a process of discovery. And doesn't every dish taste better when it comes from a playful heart? (Well, truthfully, no.) We should warn you now, this book contains kid-invented recipes. We call these "Culinary Frontiers" recipes. They're included to show you how playful children can be in the kitchen, but we can't in good conscience recommend that you actually prepare those dishes.

We realize our philosophy of cooking might require some letting go. It's true that you may not create something delicious (or even edible) each time. We hope, though, that in the process your kids become curious and enthused about food. You also might laugh with your kids, create something unexpectedly delicious, and have a

unholy combinations of ingredients and unspeakable messes, but it's also helped our kids become slightly more willing to taste something new. More important, our family has come to see food as an adventure that connects us and makes us laugh. That feels like a revelation.

Our Philosophy

In our family, cooking isn't about creating a dish that matches a picture on Instagram or sticking to a precise recipe. It's not even about making meals that satisfy every palate. It's about wel-

family adventure that makes your kitchen feel like a playground.

Mostly Fresh, Not Fancy

Just so we're all clear here: we come to this cookbook as parents rather than professional chefs. We have two young kids, so we're in the thick of it and really get the importance of simplicity and efficiency when it comes to feeding your family. While we fantasize about baking bread, growing all of our own vegetables, and sharing kale and quinoa casserole with our kids every night, that's just not how we roll in real life. We need short-cuts. Just like many American parents, we're susceptible to the charms of convenience.

You won't see any gourmet recipes or hard-to-find ingredients in this book. In our house-hold, we don't have a supply of truffle-infused butter or ground buckwheat hulls. We don't whip up Pinterest-perfect dishes or cut our kids' food into cute animal shapes. We don't braise or use a double boiler. All the dishes in this cook-book are made with easy-to-find ingredients available at most supermarkets; all can be pre-pared in less than an hour (many in half that). Our recipes never assume experience: they ap-peal to adults and kids, and they call for impro-visation. We're not into being fancy, but we are into using fresh whole foods and exploring in our kitchen-laboratory with our children. We aren't perfectionists. Sure, we believe in eating mostly fresh, real, seasonal, unprocessed ingre-dients (and we try to make that kind of eating our normal routine), but we also believe in the occasional doughnut.

We've had plenty of flops and fumbling in the food realm, but we're finding our way as a family. A celebration of the unexpected and de-lightful paths to real foods, *The Adventurous Eaters Club* shows that saying yes to kids' culi-nary impulses can make mealtime an adventure for the whole family. We hope this book in-spires your family to find your path to happy meals. Welcome to adventure-style cooking, where the focus is on joy—and healthful food is just a by-product.

Changing the way your family eats isn't easy, and there isn't one trick or rule that's going to solve it all. We've done our best to condense nuggets from the pros that have inspired us to shift our family's approach to food. We hope they inspire your family, too. No need to take all this on. Implement what works for your family, disregard what doesn't. As parents whose chil-dren now request kale salad as their comfort food on a rainy day, we're here to report: dinner with kids can be peaceful, healthy, and fun.*

---

* *Disclaimer*: Yes, our children gorge on raw cabbage and kale with-out bribery or nagging. But before you get too jealous, we should inform you that just because our kids happily eat vegetables, we should not be construed as successful parents in any broad sense. In case you're tempted to put us on a parenting pedestal, let us in-form you that our children crawl into our bed every night around 2:00 a.m. and proceed to kick us in the ribs for the remainder of the night, so any advice contained in this book was written by parents who get regularly pummeled in their sleep.

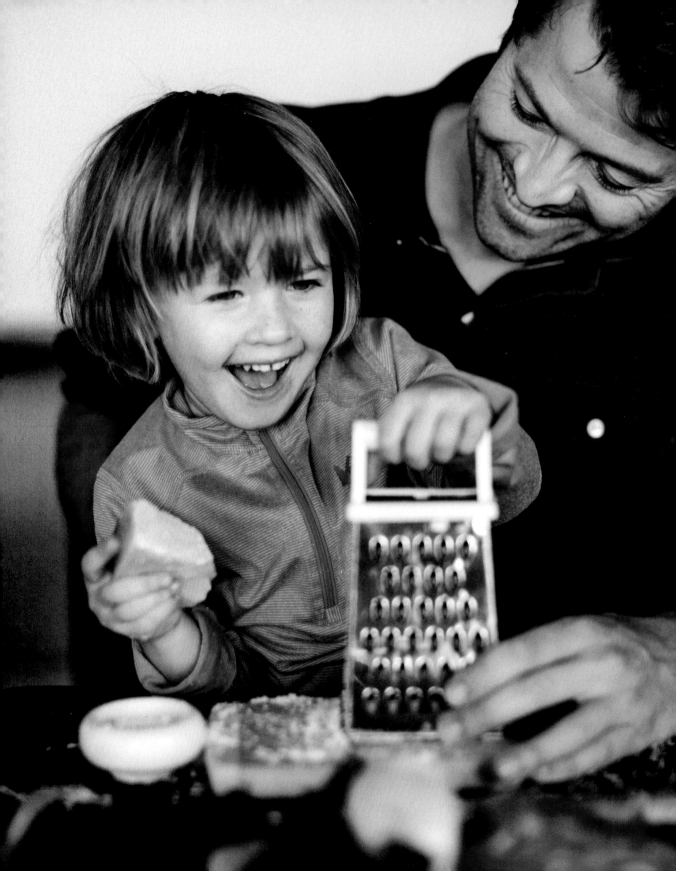

CHAPTER 2

TEN SECRETS TO HAPPY, ADVENTUROUS FAMILY MEALS

1. Welcome Kids into the Kitchen

When our son was seven years old, he and his buddy Miles took charge of making salad for a family dinner. We let them do it their way and mostly stayed out of their hair. The ingredients: romaine lettuce, kale, raw collard greens, fistfuls of fresh chives, blueberries, cucumbers, tomatoes, rosemary branches, and grated Parmesan. They topped the salad with enough lavender to stock a potpourri shop, then submerged it in several pints of dressing. Next, Miles grabbed a potato masher and pounded the greens until the veins in his neck bulged.

Once the salad had been pulverized into a drippy green pulp, Miles looked up to ask: "Does salad normally get cooked?" Okay, sometimes we let our adult biases impede culinary innovation. This was one of those times. We told him salad does not normally get cooked. Merci-fully, they opted to serve their garden puree raw. At dinner, Miles (whose parents swear he never eats salad) and West slurped down every last bit of that wet green mush, congratulating themselves on their culinary achievement. The adults had a harder time choking it down.

Of course our kids won't actually eat *everything* they make (we won't, either), but even when they won't consume their own creations, the process of combining ingredients often fuels their excitement about cooking *and* eating.

Offering our kids the chance to help cook has been central to changing our family's approach to food. Now we see the kitchen as an indoor playground of sorts (sorry, there may be a mess). We find that when our kids are involved in the cooking process, even if they're just grating cheese or peeling the garlic, they're more likely to enjoy eating the meal. They take pride in what they've helped create. Participating in meal prep gives them a chance to get to know ingredients, and the opportunity to see, smell, and touch those elements that offer a valuable sensory experience. Experts say this exposure makes kids more open to tasting new foods and our informal experiments bear this out.

If we want our kids to enjoy eating a wide range of foods, let's invite them to be part of the food-prep process. Maybe they'll create a dish that's too watery or too spicy or just plain inedible. That's okay. As long as our kids are becoming curious and excited about food, we know we're on the right track.

Aliza Miner, a chef and director of an edible schoolyard program at an elementary school in Los Angeles, is devoted to helping children expand their palates. In her school-laboratory, she's found that when her students are served a new dish that contains unfamiliar spices (such as yellow split pea dal), they won't touch it. However, when the kids help cook the meal and smell the spices in the process, they devour it.

All the recipes in this book involve some grating, washing, grinding, pounding, or other tasks that are ideally suited for young cooks, so there's always a way kids can participate. "What really struck me was how much power you can give kids in the kitchen. I always thought you needed to have an adult right there—hovering, interjecting," said Tina Hoban, who ran the early education baking program at a Montessori school in the Pacific Northwest. "Really, what I've learned by teaching cooking to young children is that you can give them some fundamentals and stand back. I really had to train myself not to be so eager to jump in and show them the best way." Although Hoban always takes the bread in and out of the oven herself, she allows her students (under eight years old) to be in charge of all the other steps in the bread-baking process.

2. Embrace the Mess

Rebels that we are, we invite you to brazenly defy Emily Post's sage advice on table manners. Even though Miss Manners wouldn't approve, play with your food. In our household, we've been known to conduct absurd taste tests, invent oddball meals, and fashion fennel fronds into facial hair. We believe play is good for kids (and parents). A friendly game of cabbage handball, for example, can give kids a valuable sensory experience with cabbage—teaching them how it smells and how it feels (and how it flies

VICKI'S KITCHEN SKILLS HAVE COME A LOOOONG WAY

My sister and I were garden-variety 1980s latchkey kids who scavenged in the freezer for a bag of peas and mooched hot meals from neighbors. We *never* sat down for dinner as a family at home. Sometimes my dad would take us to McDonald's or to the local cafeteria in my hometown. Maybe my parents subsisted on dust particles. I'm not sure, but I never saw them cook, and I learned exactly nothing about cooking from them.

When I was ten, I opened a restaurant in the basement of our home called Vicki's Health Food Palace. It was a real dive that served mustard-greens smoothies and ramen noodles smothered in a white sauce made of cream cheese, sour cream, ranch dressing, cottage cheese, and yogurt. Let's just say I didn't have a lot of repeat customers.

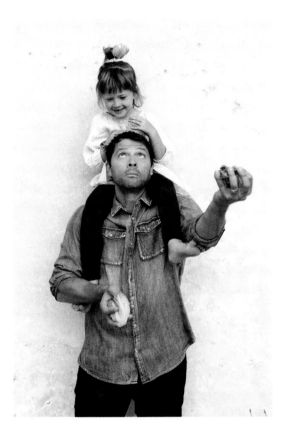
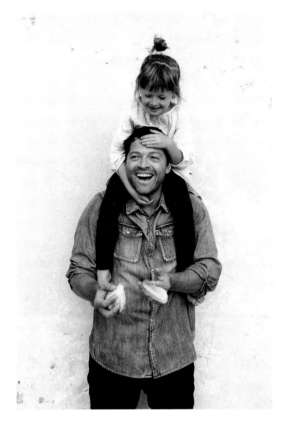

through the air). Play is an important way that children learn about everything—even food. So if our kids play with a new food on their plates, we consider that a win. It means they're getting to know a new food and will be more likely to eat it down the road.

"The purpose of the food's presence on a child's plate is for her to see it, smell it, touch it, hear it, crunch it under her fork, and perhaps taste it," according to pediatrician Nimali Fernando and pediatric feeding expert Melanie Potock, authors of *Raising a Healthy, Happy Eater*. Welcoming silliness at meals also reduces the pressure kids often feel at the table. We let

our kids eat salad with their hands, eat oatmeal with a giant serving spoon, and eat noodles with kitchen tongs. Sometimes we say, "Let's invent a breakfast that no one has ever cooked before." That play gets our kids fired up about food.

Sometimes food play gets messy. If you've ever watched a webisode of *Cooking Fast & Fresh with West*, you know that our family allows things to get messy—really, *really* messy. Bad messy. Scrub things off the ceiling messy. As parents, we'll confess, we don't find this easy; in fact, we dread it. We're burned out from the constant cleanup that young kids require, and we don't always have the time and energy to mop down the kitchen. We occasionally endure a mustard-smeared cabinet because we want our kids to feel free to experiment in the kitchen, and worrying about keeping it tidy puts a crimp in all that. Food experts say that getting messy with food is one way young kids get familiar with new foods and serves as a stepping-stone to tasting them.

3. Divide and Conquer

Who's the boss around here? Setting up some clear boundaries around food can help make mealtime more fun and peaceful for everyone. If kids (or parents) are unclear about who's in charge when it comes to eating, food-related power struggles are likely to ruin the mood. The American Academy of Pediatrics advises parents to set up a crystal clear "division of responsibility" around food—it's the gold standard for fostering a kid's healthy, happy relationship with food. When parents and kids know what they're each responsible for when it comes to food, mealtime can transform from a turf war to bonding time.

PARENTS' RESPONSIBILITY

Unless you're making a special exception, parents get to decide *what* food is served, *when* it's served, and *where* it's served. Parents are responsible for choosing which foods are bought at the store, planning the menu, making sure that everyone in the family shows up to the table for meals, and regulating the timing and content of snacks (i.e., no eating before dinner, no eating while suspended upside down on a trapeze, and so on). Once you serve dinner, though, your job is done for the duration of the meal. Sit back and trust your kids; the rest is their dominion.

KIDS' RESPONSIBILITY

Kids decide *which* of the served foods they are going to eat and *how much* they will eat. This is the kids' domain. If a parent serves peas, rice, and bug toenails (which raises an important question: do bugs have toenails?), kids get to choose which items to eat without pressure from their parents. If they decide to eat the toenails but leave the rice and peas on their plate, they might go to bed hungry. And that's the child's choice. We shared this division of responsibility with our kids—and if roles get confused, we remind them (or, more likely, they remind us). Our kids love knowing what they're in charge of. West relishes reprimanding us when we overstep, which we do . . . often.

Okay, okay, but can't we insist that our kids take just one single little bite? Many families use the "one bite" (aka the "no thank you bite") rule. Pediatric food experts say that forcing kids to take even one bite is a parental overstep. "Pickier children . . . may need as many as 32 steps before they are ready to put a food in their mouth!" writes Maryann Jacobsen, a family nutrition expert. Family therapist Ellyn Satter, the go-to international authority on pediatric eating issues, agrees: "Based on what I know about children and about feeding, let me give you my recommendation. You are obligated to provide a certain amount of food for each child. . . . No child must be forced to take—or eat—anything that she doesn't want, not even one, little, tiny almost invisible bite." Forcing an anxious eater to eat even one tiny bite can intensify the child's anxiety around food, which decreases appetite and intensifies picky eating. A kid with permission *not* to eat is more likely to feel comfortable trying something new.

What if you have a kid who's so easily distracted that sometimes she's more likely to braid the placemat fringe than consume lunch? (We have a kid like that.) While the pros advise against pressuring kids to eat, they say it's okay to encourage kids to tune in to their own bodies at mealtime: "Are you full or still hungry? What does your tummy say?" Sometimes we ask, "Want to try the cauliflower?" We don't insist they try it, but we might remind them that it's there for them to try if they're daydreaming.

4. Ditch the Grazing Habit

Many children in the US snack all day long—and the majority of these snacks are highly processed, carb-heavy foods like crackers, chips, and baked goods.

The more insidious downside of all-day snacking is that it perpetuates the habit of eating a limited diet of familiar beige foods. While studies show that kids are fully capable of learning to love new foods (including fresh produce), they'll happily stick to a diet of Goldfish crackers if they're snacking whenever they please.

Kid-food experts suggest something simple . . . eat only at set meal and snack times, and leave at least *two hours* between snacks and meals. This means our kids will likely feel hungry at mealtime—which is exactly what we want. Hunger is a perfectly human sensation, and it's healthy for children to experience it in small doses. (We're not talking about the tragedy of starvation that too many children around the world face.) The occasional hunger pain allows kids to tune in to their bodies, learn about the flow of sensations in their stomachs, and develop the fine art of patience. If we feed kids only at fixed meal and snack times, they'll show up for meals hungry (ideally, not freaking-out-biting-other-children hungry) and be more likely to eat a variety of foods.

If your kids are used to eating whenever they want, it'll take some parental resolve to shift to designated meal and snack times. Here's a quick guide to how often kids need to eat, depending on their ages (barring any medical issues):

Toddlers need to eat every two to three hours: three meals, three snacks.

Preschool-age kids: three meals, two snacks.

School-age children: three meals, one snack.

OUR FAMILY SNACK CONTRACT

We'll eat three meals per day at roughly these times: _____

We'll eat _____ snacks per day at roughly these times: _____

If you're making the switch from free-range grazing to set mealtimes, announce the new policy to the family (i.e., no eating between planned meals and snacks) so they know what's coming. When your kid asks for food at a nonscheduled time, hold the line: "I know you'd love to have a cookie right now, but we're not going to eat now because we're having dinner in an hour." No need to deliver a compelling lecture. Just don't cave to the kids' panhandling for food between meals or outside the designated snack time.

Instead of letting kids graze, serve the snack and get your kids to the table to eat it. Remove the snack plate when they leave the table, or after fifteen or twenty minutes, so they stop snacking long before mealtime. If the snack plate stays out, they'll keep on snacking till dinner.

ADVENTUROUS KID EATERS SAY...

KIANA, AGE SEVEN

What I'm most excited to taste: Pig brains, when we go to Thailand for vacation.

What I'm most afraid to eat: Scorpions. Duh.

My advice to kids who are afraid to try new foods: If you try it, you might like it. If not, if you try again, you'll probably like it. That happened to me with green beans, broccoli, and especially spinach. The first times I ate it, I did not like it at *all*. Now I usually have spinach with butter and salt; it's actually pretty tasty.

I like to eat: Fish, crab, salmon, clams, seaweed (not straight off the beach—I like it dried), hot sauce, jalapeño-flavored chips, spinach, and broccoli (the stump is actually sweet!).

My signature dish: I invented my own mac 'n' cheese recipe. It has salt and pepper, green onions, and a bunch of spices. I love green onions in my mac 'n' cheese.

5. Children (Yes, Even Yours) Can Love Real Food

Our children have had plenty of exposure to seafood since we moved to the coastal Pacific Northwest. Ever since preschool, West and Maison have spent their summers hoisting up rocks on the beach to watch tiny crabs scurry. When we go out crabbing as a family, West is always the first to reach his bare hands into the crab trap to wrestle out snapping adult crabs.

Come summer, it's not unusual for us to receive SOS texts from friends and neighbors who have hauled in fresh Dungeness crab in the bay: "EMERGENCY, caught too much crab, want some?" The answer is *always*: yes, please. The adults in our family swoon over fresh crab.

When asked if our kids ate crab, however, we'd have to admit that they hadn't even tried it. If you know anything about the Pac Northwest food scene, you realize how very uncool this is. Whenever we'd sit down to feast on steamy fresh Dungeness, our kids would subtly scooch their chairs away from the table. We tried every ill-advised pressure tactic we could think of, including chiding them, "Do you know how lucky we are to have fresh crab?! It's delicious. Try it!" Our pestering did absolutely nothing to inspire our kids to taste it. We eventually gave up. We tried to focus on enjoying our steaming fresh catch at the family meal while our kids nibbled on grilled corn on the cob.

After a mere *four years* of catching crab and watching us feast on them, West asked us to describe the flavor of crab. He said he was considering tasting it but wanted more info. After some hemming and hawing, we realized we didn't have a decent parallel. What compares to crab texture or flavor? We were stumped. "The flavor isn't fishy. It's salty," Misha mustered. West mulled it over for a few weeks. Then one night he went for it—a fresh crab claw dipped in melted butter. He went back for seconds. Not wanting to get one-upped by her big brother, Maison followed and took her first bite at the same meal— she looked surprised and said, "Not bad." We tried to keep our poker faces on, but inside we were both bursting with the glow of sweet victory.

Kids can take a long time to warm up to an unfamiliar food; teaching them to eat new foods calls for a truly unreasonable amount of patience. "The way you teach a child to eat well is through example, enthusiasm, and patient exposure to good food," writes food historian Bee Wilson, author of *First Bite*. Young children naturally distrust anything new or different, so we can't expect them to instantly devour our buttered snails. After one or two attempts, parents in the US often give up and conclude, "My kid would never eat that." Studies show that approximately one-quarter of parents in the US think their children dislike a food after serving it only twice.

In fact, it can take preschoolers *ten to fifteen* exposures to a new food before they're willing to taste it—and even more exposures before they accept and enjoy it. Susan Roberts, Tufts University nutritionist and coauthor of *Feeding Your Child for Lifelong Health*, suggests putting a new food on the table fifteen times to give kids the chance to try it and learn to like it. Encourage kids to taste a new food, but if the kid doesn't want it, don't make a fuss—just remove it and try again another time. And another time after that. And another time after that. Patience, young Padawan, patience.

To make matters trickier, at age two or three, kids enter a developmental phase called neophobia, when they become especially fearful

of new foods. This food phase can last several *years*. (The French call this stage *la phase d'opposition*. Leave it to the French to make something super annoying sound cool.) During this phase, kids might stop eating some foods they previously liked, become resistant to anything they see as new or different, and become more sensitive to environmental eating cues.

During this window of time, American parents often begin to believe that their kids are incapable of eating anything new and begin serving a limited selection of familiar kids foods. But food pros suggest that parents not get discouraged during this phase and continue to expose kids to a wide variety of foods. (See page 263, where we've listed more strategies for eating meals with toddlers.)

In addition, it should be noted that toddlers have maddeningly erratic eating habits. They consume lots of food one day and seem to subsist on air the next. They devour a particular food one minute, eschew it the next. So when a kid isn't eating a meal, instead of tensing up and offering cereal as a knee-jerk reaction, remember that toddler eating habits are wild, and their intake fluctuates. Remember that tastes are learned and almost all children are capable of learning to love diverse foods.

6. Baby Steps: Mix It Up

When planning a family dinner, focus on what *you* want to eat—let variety, adventure, and pleasure inform your choices. Consider not having the same main dish more than once a week. While the pros advise not catering to kids' limited tastes, it's helpful to take kids' preferences into account when preparing dinner and letting them weigh in. If a kid asks for rice with chicken one night, you could make rice if you haven't been eating rice every day that week. Or you could say, "We had rice last night. Tonight we're having noodles. Do you want curly or straight?"

We can't expect children to make the leap from chicken nuggets to pâté in one day—or even in one month. Think baby steps. Be strategic with your meal planning. On nights that you're serving a main dish that's new or that you already know isn't your kid's favorite, include two or three "safe foods" in the meal as well. If kids see something familiar on their plates,

they'll likely feel more relaxed and less pressured, which may lead them to taste something new. "While you don't want kids to dictate the menu, you also want them to look down at their plate and see something that is familiar," writes family nutrition expert Maryann Jacobsen.

At meals, present kids with small amounts of a few different options, and allow them to choose which items they want to eat. For example, offer a make-your-own salad bar with a range of fresh ingredients. Don't evaluate or comment on their choices. Kids can choose what (and how much) to eat from what's been offered at the meal. If a kid wants more of something, let her have more.

One way to tiptoe toward new foods is to use what experts call food bridges. Start with flavors and textures your child already enjoys, and use them as a "bridge" to a new food. For example, if a kid likes cheese but hasn't been ready to try broccoli, explore broccoli topped with melted cheese as a bridge.

One bridge-building strategy is to slightly modify a kid's favorite dish. If a child likes French toast, cut and cook the bread the usual way, but invite your kid to add a new spice to the egg mixture—perhaps a sprinkle of nutmeg. Or if your kid loves spaghetti, get her involved in adding something new to it (fresh spinach?), or keep the pasta sauce the same and just try a new pasta shape (gasp) . . . like bow ties. This might be a stretch for some kids. Newness can be scary—and exciting. Just one small change to a familiar food can open new possibilities.

Talk about the bridge. When your kid meets a new food with clenched teeth, talk about the similarities between the new food and foods he already knows and accepts. Example: "You know how you liked that quiche with zucchini? This omelet has zucchini in it." (Sure, these

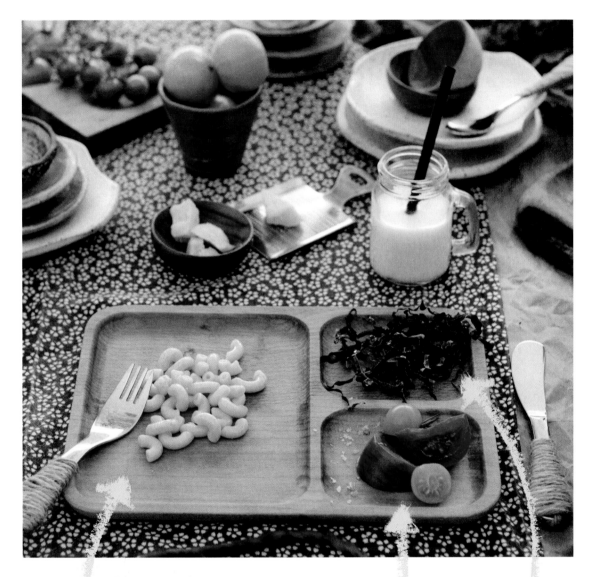

Serve tiny, taste-safe portions.
Serve two known foods and one new food.

New Food

Familiar/Accepted Food

Familiar/Accepted Food

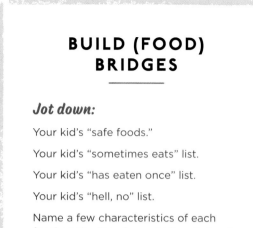

BUILD (FOOD) BRIDGES

Jot down:

Your kid's "safe foods."

Your kid's "sometimes eats" list.

Your kid's "has eaten once" list.

Your kid's "hell, no" list.

Name a few characteristics of each food on the list of your kid's safe foods. Crunchy or smooth? Savory or sweet? Salty or cheesy? Dry or wet?

Brainstorm foods with similar characteristics.

might be boring conversations, but they can be useful for kids learning to brave new foods.)

Encourage kids to use words like *crunchy*, *salty*, and *melty* instead of *good* and *bad* to help pinpoint why a food feels or tastes good in the mouth. When offering a new food, use those same words to bridge the gap. Example: "This feta cheese is crumbly like the sausage you like—and salty, too." Instead of singing the praises of this new food, which could feel like pressure, simply describe the similarities between accepted, known foods and the new food.

7. One Family, One Meal (No Short-Order Cooking)

Instead of preparing a separate "kid-friendly" meal for children, prepare one meal for the en-tire family. Stop asking your child, "What do you want to eat for dinner tonight?" Instead, decide what's for dinner based on a balanced, varied menu for the week. This is your purview, parents—not the kids' choice. The good news: as the parent, you cook the meals *you* want to eat. If you want to eat asparagus for dinner, cook it and serve it. Keep cooking it, even if your kids think they don't like it. After a while, they'll see you eating it, they'll see it on their plates, they might someday muster the nerve to touch it with a fork (and find that they don't instantly turn into toads), and eventually they might eat it right alongside you.

That's the long game anyway. Along the way, there will likely be some challenges. If your young 'uns are used to dictating what's for dinner or getting their own specialized meals, it'll take some parental fortitude to transition into a new way of eating together.

The scenario: you're serving a family dinner of salad, chicken, and rice. Your kid responds, "I really want a grilled cheese!" and refuses to eat *anything* on her plate. Naturally, panic sets in immediately. You start to spin . . . *Will she be too hungry to sleep? Will she hate me for starving her? Am I setting the stage for eating disorders down the road? I'm a horrible parent. Why didn't I just serve grilled cheese for dinner? Will she murder me in my sleep?*

Do you . . .

a. Force her to stay at the table until she consumes three bites

b. Insist she clean her plate

c. Quickly make her a grilled cheese

d. Lecture her about how good for her the dinner is and how hard you worked to prepare it *e.* Threaten to take away her dessert

f. Promise her cake if she eats two bites of dinner

g. Freak out about how stressful family meals are

When your child refuses the meal you've prepared, it may seem like no big deal to jump up to whip up a grilled cheese. But here's the thing: if you serve a backup special kids' meal, you're sending a very clear message that kids will absorb—that they don't have to learn to eat anything they aren't familiar with.

"In many families, parents announce dinner and kids protest. Then parents get anxious that the kid won't eat enough and back down by asking the child what they would like to eat. When a parent asks the child what she'd like, it puts the child in the inappropriate role of choosing food for the family. Kids don't have the knowledge necessary to make such important choices," according to the nutrition guide for parents published by the American Academy of Pediatrics. When parents provide an alternative meal, this puts the child in charge of the menu, which disrupts the appropriate food roles for parents and children (in sum: parents should provide the meal, and children should decide what and how much to eat from what's offered).

If we want our families to eat a variety of foods but our kids demand pizza for the third night in a row, we can facilitate this by holding firm. Experts suggest a response like this: "You don't have to eat it if you don't want to, but this is what we're having for dinner tonight. We'll have pizza again soon." Don't give a rousing speech on why she should eat the meal you've lovingly prepared. Don't pressure her to eat. And don't prepare a backup meal. "Children are clever. They know when we will give in. . . .

If you cave and give them other meals, they will surely repeat the performance next mealtime," writes Dreena Burton, chef and mother of three. "This doesn't mean force your children to eat one particular food they really don't like (i.e., eggplant) or eat everything on their plate. . . . But if they know you are in the habit of giving in and allowing them to have something else, they'll hold out until you do!"

This is tricky for parents. If our kid doesn't eat a thing at dinner and we don't provide a backup special meal, our kid might leave the table hungry. Yikes. We find this really tough—somehow the mere thought of allowing our kids to be hungry even for a few hours feels wrong. "You probably worry that if your child doesn't eat, she'll get hungry. Of course, she will! And when she's hungry, she'll eat. . . . If your toddler misses a meal of her own free choice, it won't make her sick and she'll probably be ready to eat at the next regular meal or snack time," according to the American Academy of Pediatrics' nutrition guide for parents.

The other thing that really trips parents up when they ponder giving their kids the freedom to not eat, is the prospect of wasted food. Considering that so many children around the world don't have enough to eat and the appalling quantity of food waste in America, this is a righteous concern. Parents in the US often cite food-waste concern as a reason for not serving children new foods. After all, why serve broccoli if your kid won't eat it? Stress over food waste can set off a cycle of guilt and tension around food that can have a lasting impact on kids. Ideally, we'd be able to let our kids eat—or not—without feeling judged. If we don't offer our kids a new or challenging food because we're afraid it'll get wasted, we're missing the opportunity to expand our kids' willingness to eat a range of foods.

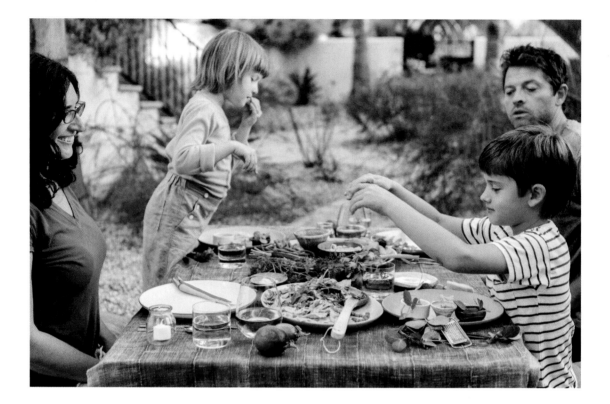

To minimize waste, serve your kids *tiny* portions of new foods. Also, as parents, we're allowed to eat our kids' leftovers. You know how we steal french fries off our kids' plates? The same rule applies to leftover broccoli, so there's no excuse to stop serving vegetables. Plus, eating more whole fresh foods as a family means consuming less plastic and packaging.

8. Keep Your Cool and Pull the Plug on the Power Struggle

You've had a long day, then you prepare a healthful dinner for your family. Your kid asks: "What are you cooking?" "Chicken cacciatore," you respond. Your kid distorts her face, throws herself on the floor, writhes as if in pain, and starts yelling, *"Yuck! Bleck!"* She's never had chicken cacciatore, but she won't even consider trying it.

You might be really, really tempted to lecture about healthful eating. You might want to beg, cajole, or bribe. Or yell, "Eat it, you ungrateful monster!" Or throw up your hands and prepare that backup grilled cheese. Halt.

When kids get attention around refusing food, the struggle gains them power. To neutralize it, experts say, it's best to stop reacting, stop engaging with it. (Yep, this can be a challenge.) So if your kid says, *"Ewwww.* Yuck! I don't like cauliflower!" here's how the experts suggest responding:

- "That's okay. You don't have to eat anything you don't want to. There's plenty of other food to eat."
- "That's okay. You haven't tasted it enough times yet. We'll try another time." Or "Maybe you'll like it when you're more grown up."
- Share the "Don't yuck my yum" rule. Let your kid know that it's fine to say, "No, thank you," and it's fine to choose not to eat something, but it's not okay to say, "That's disgusting."
- Just remove the offending food from the plate without comment.
- Resist the temptation to give your kid a lecture on how hard you worked to prepare the meal.
- Don't pressure, coerce, cajole, threaten, or bribe, and don't herald the health benefits.
- Give your kid some context for the food if it's something new and she didn't help you cook it. Example: "This is cauliflower. I used to eat it as a kid in Germany. It tastes a little like broccoli." Use neutral words to describe the food.
- Eat your own dinner, enjoy it, and change the subject. Talk about anything other than food!

The French seem to have food figured out. "Opposition to food can't persist if there is no opponent. In the face of a child's refusal to eat, the best parental response is serene indifference. Parents should remind themselves . . . my child will not continue refusing to eat if I simply refuse to react," according to one classic French parenting book. From the French point of view, very few foods actually taste bad, so a child's aversion to food is more psychological than physiological. If a French kid isn't game to try olives, the parents don't make a fuss or force it—they also don't remove olives from the menu because a kid has refused them. They understand that it takes time and repeated exposure for kids to accept and enjoy a new food, so they just keep serving olives.

9. Don't Pass On Your Bad Habits

In modern American culture, many of us are stressed about feeding our kids—and kids feel it. Anxiety, tension, and anything that children perceive as pressure decreases appetite. Being playful and having fun can relax kids (and parents), which in turn makes everyone more likely to enjoy eating and tasting unfamiliar foods. And as cheesy as this may sound, research also shows that children are more likely to try a food they think they dislike when it's presented by a smiling adult.

That's all well and good, but it's not easy to smile and enjoy mealtime, when you have an anxiety-ridden relationship with food, which many of us do. Whether we're caught up in the latest micronutrients, diet trends, or nutrition and health fads, Americans tend to have particularly "complicated" relationships with food. That's because most of us are trying to lose weight. Between one-third and one-half of adults in the US surveyed said they were dieting to lose or maintain weight. In 2017, the weight-loss industry was worth more than $66 billion per year in the US alone. In 2000, the American Dietetic Association found that 40 percent of Americans feel conflicted or anxious about their food choices. Many of us are embroiled in a constant state of angst regarding food—we're eating too much gluten, not

MEAL PLANNING CLIFFSNOTES

- Set the menu according to what you, the parent, want to eat rather than catering to kids' limited culinary repertoire.
- Keep exposing kids to new foods, even if they don't like them at first.
- Remember that taste is learned and your kid can learn to like new foods if you set a structure that supports that.
- Offer some familiar foods alongside an unfamiliar food.
- Serve tiny portions so kids don't get overwhelmed (they can always have more).
- Put variety, adventure, and joy at the top of your meal-planning agenda.
- Build food bridges to help kids venture into new foods.

enough protein, too much sugar, or too few antioxidants.

Restricted eating has become so ingrained in American culture that it's hard for us to imagine another way. "Regular attempts to eat less than we are really hungry for or to settle for less appealing food than we really want, has," according to the go-to pediatric feeding authority Ellyn Satter, "become such a fixed part of our relationship with food that it's hard for most people to see that the negativity and restraint around food are anything but normal. They are not."

This restrained, worry-laden eating style affects the way we feed our children. If parents are anxious and worried about food, their children tend to pick up on it.

While Americans tend to be anxious about food and focus on health, nutrition, and dieting, the French think about food very differently. Highlighting this culture gap, when Americans were shown a picture of chocolate cake, they most commonly used the word *guilt*, while the French used the word *celebration*. In spite of the way the French embrace food, the obesity rate for French children is among the lowest in the developed world. The US ranks at the top.

Although American culture tends to cycle through health fads, the director of Yale University's Prevention Research Center says that what constitutes a healthful diet isn't a mystery: "A diet of minimally processed foods close to nature, predominantly plants, is decisively associated with health promotion." Moreover, eating a *variety* of foods tends to lead to greater health.

We know that processed foods aren't healthful per se, but when we're talking to our kids about food, let's focus on joy and permission rather than demonizing particular foods. Labeling a certain food "bad" or making it taboo isn't helpful anyway—it tends to increase a kid's preference for it. Even the "eating clean" trend, which urges us to eliminate flour, sugar, and processed foods, can feel like a lot of restriction to a kid who really wants a cookie—and when cookies are verboten, they're way more likely to become the focus of attention. Likewise, giving them a spiel on the health benefits of spinach is totally ineffective in persuading them to eat it. Sure, some foods are better than others at nourishing the body, but foods have different purposes. Sometimes there's emotional or celebratory value in eating something that isn't particularly healthful, like cake and ice cream on your birthday.

Parents have a major impact on kids' food preferences. We can do our best not to saddle our kids with our grown-up food issues by keeping our personal dietary restrictions under wraps so that our kids don't take them on. As parents, we can help our kids pry open their taste buds or we can shut down their willingness to try new foods by imposing our own culinary judgments on them. Once when Maison was wolfing down some salty seaweed, a friend asked to try some. The kid's mother scrunched up her face and said, "Really? You can try it if you want. I find it so fishy tasting." Reading her mom's response, the five-year-old changed her mind and never tried the salty, crispy treat that Maison relishes. She missed an opportunity to taste something new.

Instead of imposing our judgments on whether a food is "good" or "bad," what if we bring a spirit of exploration and celebration to the way we eat with our families? That doesn't mean allowing our families to eat cake at every meal. But worrying about healthy food and concentrating on restricting sugar intake doesn't lead us to a joyful relationship with food. When you're tempted to obsess over eliminating certain foods from your family's diet, try shifting your focus to the fun you can have discovering new, diverse dishes together. Food can be a wondrous adventure for the whole family, when we approach it with openness and curiosity. This brings us to our final, most important family food principle.

10. Convivialité = Happy Meals

The French are experts at enjoying food. Teaching children to "taste everything" is a top priority for French parents and teachers—who consider learning to savor food as important as learning to read and to subtract. French parents don't focus on teaching kids how to eat healthy food; they focus on what they think kids most need to learn about food—namely, how to savor and enjoy it.

Whether settling in for supper in Lyon, or waking up to croissants and fresh fruit in Provence, mealtimes in France revolve around the principle of *convivialité*, which means something like feasting or socializing together. The French approach to food puts pleasure at the

> *What some call health, if purchased by perpetual anxiety about diet, isn't much better than a tedious disease.*
> —GEORGE DENNISON PRENTICE

center of the experience. When we're worrying about counting calories or keeping score of the micronutrients we've consumed, it's hard to enjoy food. How might we bring more *convivialité* to our meals?

Our family has found its own way to bring more joy to eating together. We like to devise family challenges like: Can we make a family meal that's totally green without using any artificial coloring? Can we find a vegetable that no one in our family has tried and sample it together? These tasks get our children inspired to cook and eat.

Bring on the *Convivialité*

LET MEALS BE A HAPPY PAUSE

Many parents find family meals stressful. You probably don't need us to tell you that arguing about food is not fun. At all. If family meals have been tense, switch up your mealtime rituals to reset the vibe. Is there something that might make meals feel more relaxing and fun? How about putting away cell phones, iPads, and anything that beeps and/or whistles? We're not proposing anything complicated or time consuming. Often there is a simple way to make meals feel like a happy pause. Our chil-

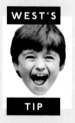

WEST'S TIP

Kids can set the table, fold napkins, pour drinks, clean the table, and pick flowers from the garden. How do you like to set the table in your home? Can you draw a picture of it? Is there something you'd like to add to the place settings to make dinner special tonight?

dren's school asks them to eat lunch in silence for five minutes every day. (We haven't yet been able to master this at home.) Even setting the table, lighting a candle, putting some flowers out, or changing up the conversation can make meals a happier experience with more connection.

MEALTIME CONVERSATION STARTERS

Instead of focusing on what kids are (or aren't) eating, focus mealtime conversation on topics that have nothing to do with food. There's nothing wrong with starting with a basic question about everyone's day. Maison likes to give a de-

tailed account of her activities, then she asks us to do the same. Try these family conversation starters:

- The funniest thing that happened today.
- Something you learned today.
- Something you did to help someone today.
- Something kind you did today.
- Your favorite summer activity.
- Which new person would you like to have as a friend?
- What's the best and worst thing about your position in the family birth order?
- Who can make you feel better when you're sad or angry?
- What special talent would you like to have?
- Is it more fun to be a parent or a child?
- What do children know more about than adults?

Adventurous Eaters Club Family Food Guidelines

Between the ages of six months and eighteen years, your children will share approximately 6,205 dinners with you, so you have ample opportunity to connect over meals. Based on expert suggestions, we created some guidelines aimed to bring more fun and connection to our family meals. We aren't a rule-loving family, but we found that having a few nonnegotiables made things easier because they help reduce bargaining and impulsiveness. Some of these are hard rules, and others serve to inspire us and remind us of who we want to be. These guidelines haven't miraculously solved all the food tensions in our household, but we find that our dining room table is more peaceful (and more fun) now that we've created some simple principles around food. We think of them as routines, customs, and habits rather than strict regulations. Here they are:

1. Welcome kids into the kitchen! Cook together, improvise, and let joy lead.

2. Play with food, make a mess in the kitchen, and clean it up together after.

3. Savor and enjoy. Create a happy atmosphere and eat meals together at the table without distractions. (We also eat in the car, because we're Americans who spend way too much time driving around, but usually we don't eat while we're hovering over the sink, watching TV, or doing headstands.)

4. Everyone eats the same meal. Translation: no special kids' meals.

5. Kids: you get to choose what and how much to eat from your plate. You don't have to eat anything you don't want to. It's not okay to call any food gross; a simple "no, thanks" will do.

6. Parents: keep your cool and stick to your lane. Don't cajole, pressure, bribe, threaten, reward, or coerce kids to eat anything. Don't even comment on what kids are or aren't eating. Deep cleansing breath.

7. Be food adventurers together—taste something new and eat a variety of foods. We try not to eat the same main dish more than once per week. This encourages us to eat variety. Be patient and keep exposing kids to new foods—even if they're not ready to try them. This process takes *time*.

8. Eat mostly whole, unprocessed foods.

9. Parents decide which food comes into the home and what's on the menu.

10. Eat at scheduled meal and snack times (without eating much in between). Think of snacks as mini meals, and stick to designated snack times.

11. Create a family food culture. Ours is: "We are food adventurers."

NOTE: We haven't read much expert advice on this, but we also found another rule to be exceptionally helpful in our household: "No one is allowed to climb or walk on the dining-room table." Yes, we had to create a rule about this.

DESIGNING YOUR OWN FAMILY FOOD GUIDELINES

Design your own family food guidelines. Ours won't work for every family. Create guidelines that will work for your family's unique schedule, circumstances, and style. Explain the new deal to your kids. It might be tricky to stick to the guidelines at first—but if you all hang in there, you might find cooking and eating more peaceful and joyful for the whole family. What are your family food values? What are your family rules around food? Create your own. Get silly and get serious.

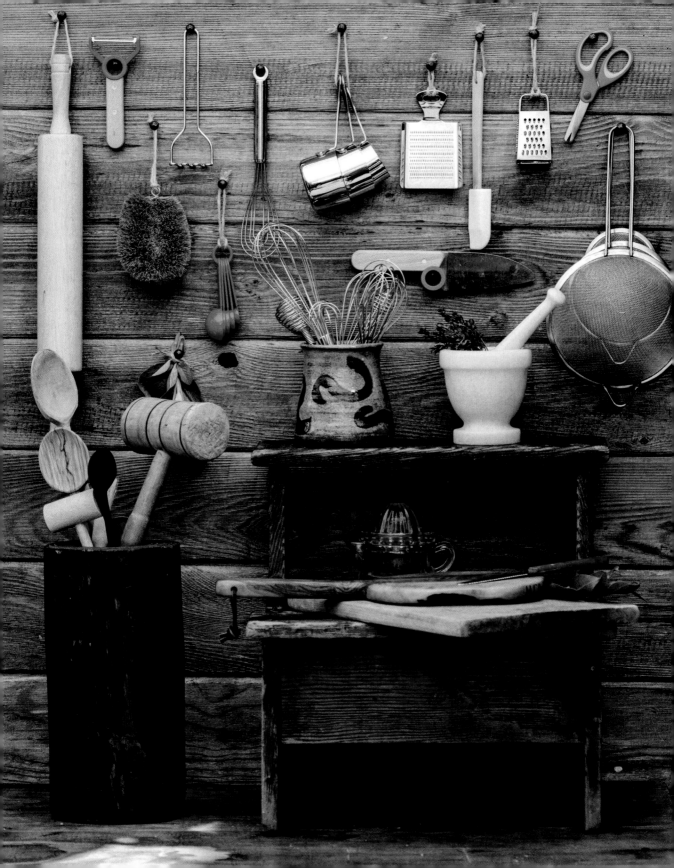

CHAPTER 3

TOOLS FOR ADVENTUROUS YOUNG CHEFS

THE KEY TO cultivating joyful, adventurous eaters is to put kids to work in the kitchen. Most kitchen equipment isn't built for tiny hands, so the more kid-size tools, the better. We have a special drawer chock-full of children's cooking utensils. Everything in it is *real*, and it works (yes, even knives).

Every recipe in this book calls for some smashing, grating, peeling, washing, or juicing, so there's always a way for kids to get their hands dirty. Even if you're short on time and aren't up for a mess tornado, there are plenty of simple ways to invite your children to participate.

Kids' Tools: The Essentials

Mini kitchen tools can be found in dollar stores, hardware stores, the baking-supplies aisle in grocery stores, and specialized online catalogs. See page 259 for suggestions about where you can stock up.

A GREAT KIDS' KNIFE: Yes, a real one. Chopping and slicing are crucial to cooking, and with the right supervision, kids can learn to use knives safely. Children as young as eighteen months are given knives in the Montessori curriculum, which focuses on fostering independence. Montessori teachers use a slow and fully supervised process for teaching kids knife skills, starting with a butter knife and eventually graduating to a small serrated knife. At first we were hesitant to let our kids cut anything, but we bought some kids' knives from an educational catalog and taught our kids how to be careful. Now they cherish—and respect—their "special" knives and take pride in using them safely. We should mention that it's *very important* to teach kids that the sharp adult knives are totally off-limits. (If you can keep them out of reach, even better.)

SMALL AND LARGE WOODEN CUTTING BOARDS: There's nothing like a nice wooden surface for chopping. Brightly colored plastic ones may be tempting, but they can hold on to germs.

MORTAR AND PESTLE: West and Maison are always game to use the mortar and pestle. They'll happily grind anything from nuts to spices to lint balls.

Food pioneer Alice Waters noted that she got her daughter interested in a variety of foods by enlisting her help in the kitchen at a young age: "She really loved pounding things in a mortar and pestle. . . . While I was doing other things, she'd pound the garlic or the basil, smelling it all at the same time." Although pounding ingredients that don't require it may seem frivolous, it offers kids an important opportunity to get to know the smell of new foods (which ultimately makes them feel more comfortable tasting new stuff), so let your kid *pound* and *grind*.

NUTCRACKERS, MALLETS, POTATO MASHERS, ROLLING PINS, AND OTHER ESSENTIAL TOOLS FOR SMASHING AND PULVERIZING: To be totally up front, mashing is a cornerstone of our family cooking "technique." This cookbook calls for a *lot* of smashing. A nice little wooden mallet can work wonders when a kid is trying to annihilate pecans or cardamom pods or pumpkin seeds. Our kids love snacking on raw nuts, and getting the shells off is a part of the charm. West prefers using a hammer to crack nuts, so that might be all you need. Still, we like to keep nutcrackers around. Mini rolling pins also make useful tools for crushing stuff. Just load your seeds or nuts into a zip-lock bag, squeeze out the air, seal, and whack with a rolling pin or slowly roll the pin over the bag.

MANUAL CITRUS PRESS (LARGE) AND KID-SIZE GLASS JUICER: Juicing is a simple and fun way for even the youngest kids to participate. Little hands are perfect for squeezing limes, tangerines, and other juicy little citruses.

GRATERS (BIG AND SMALL): Our kids love to grate pretty much anything and everything: Parmesan cheese, red cabbage, carrots, apples—you name it, they'll grate it. We keep a few kid-size box graters on hand as well as some Microplane zesters when we need to zest an orange or a lemon. Zesters have easy-to-grip handles that make them fun to use for the heck of it; they also yield a finer zest than box graters do. In our house, we let our kids use them interchangeably (gasp!) based on their moods. Some days, they're itching to make Parmesan snow—that's when a zester comes in handy (or the tiniest holes on a box grater). Other days, when we're looking to shred some cabbage, we might encourage them to use the medium holes on the box grater. It's a highly scientific process in our household. We taste as we go. How does cabbage grated with medium holes compare in crunchiness to zested cabbage? Which one makes a more fetching purple mustache?

VEGGIE PEELERS: West *loves* peeling potatoes, carrots, and cucumbers. Sure, the pros might say the Y peeler is hands down the peeler of choice. (More power! Sharper blades!) But West loves the swivel peeler. If your kid isn't totally in love with your peeler, take a stroll around your neighborhood with a fistful of carrots. Test your neighbors' peelers.

SALAD SPINNER: We hate wet lettuce. The key to beautiful salad is truly dry greens that the dressing can cling to. Unless you're going to hang your greens to dry on a sunny laundry line

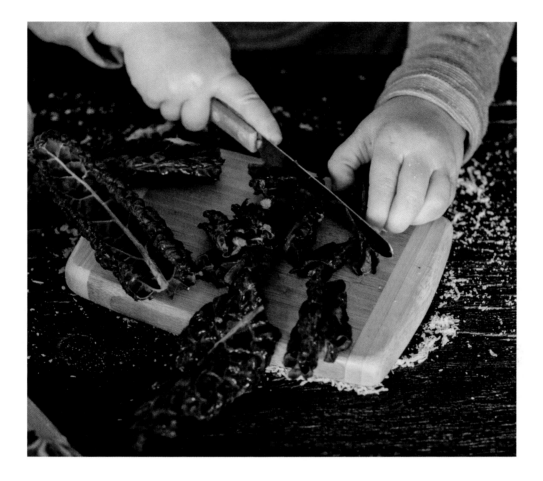

LEARN THE "CLAW" CUTTING TECHNIQUE!

Curl all your fingers and your thumb so that your hand looks like a bear claw. Growl like an angry bear. Keep the bear-claw shape with your hand and go to your cutting board. Rest the tips of your fingers on top of whatever food you're about to cut. Your fingertips should be perpendicular to the surface of the food so that your fingernails act as a shield. Then pick up the knife with your other hand—start off with a butter knife. Grip the knife on the handle, wrapping all your fingers around the knife handle. Make sure the sharp side of the blade is facing down. Keep your eagle eyes on your knife. Now press down on the knife carefully, cutting straight down rather than with a sawing motion.

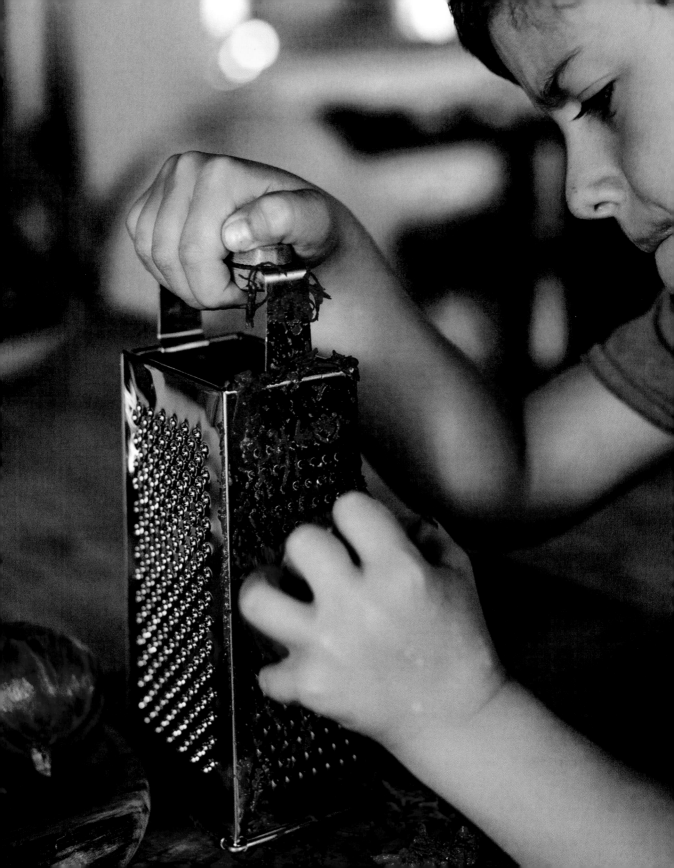

(we sometimes do), might we suggest a salad spinner? Pumping that salad spinner = pure bliss for our kids.

MEASURING CUPS AND SPOONS: Sometimes we like to be precise; sometimes we use a pinch or a handful.

KID-SIZE STEP STOOLS: We keep some short, simple two-step wooden step stools in the kitchen so the kids can always reach the counter. (Note: this can be one of those mixed blessings . . .)

CHILD SCISSORS: West and Maison love harvesting fresh herbs and snipping leafy greens. And the rounded tip means nobody gets hurt.

COLANDERS AND SIEVES: Perfect for washing berries, straining pasta, or wearing as helmets.

VEGGIE BRUSHES: We use these to scrub especially dirty root vegetables like carrots, beets, and potatoes. Remember: cool water, no soap.

POT HOLDERS: We keep a supply of big and small pot holders.

APRONS (ADULT AND KID SIZES): You have to make peace with some mess when you're cooking with kids, but there's no shame in offering aprons for all the chefs in the family. Plus, aprons can give kids the feeling of officially belonging in the kitchen.

ASSORTED SMALL HAND TOOLS: Tongs, spatulas, whisks, basting brushes, wooden spoons, and anything that can be used to mash or smash. We let our kids choose their tools for various meal-prep tasks. Sometimes they choose the least efficient tool for the job. Sometimes they serve salad with a whisk and a chopstick. Hey, it's this kind of innovation that leads to . . .

Kids' Tools: Bonus Items

Generally, we aren't into stockpiling extra kitchen gadgets, but we've found that these have helped inspire our kids to cook.

PIZZA CUTTER: Besides cutting pizza, this tool lets kids customize cookie-dough shapes and even "ribbonize" greens like kale and basil.

BANANA SLICER, EGG SLICER, APPLE SLICER: Do bananas really need their own dedicated slicing implement? Absolutely not, but West and Maison use theirs nearly every day.

APPLE PEELER/CORER/SPIRALIZER: This device attaches to a table, and we use it to peel, core, and spiral-slice apples when we're making applesauce, baked apples, or apple chips in the fall. Necessary, no. Fun, yes.

KIDS IN THE KITCHEN

Both the American Heart Association and the Mayo Clinic agree that getting children involved in grocery shopping and food prep leads to eating nutritious foods. A Columbia University study of six hundred kids found that children who helped cook their own meals were more likely to eat them. In other words, a kid who has chopped up a radish is more likely to eat a radish.

KITCHEN
SAFETY

We all know there are plenty of hazards lurking in the kitchen. The trick is to invite your children to participate without being stressed out. Here are a few basic safety guidelines we cook by:

- Always have a grown-up sous chef in the kitchen. If you have to answer the door or go to the bathroom, bring the kids with you—just don't leave them unattended in the proximity of knives and hot stoves.

- Take your time and concentrate. Rushing can be risky when there are blenders and flames nearby.

Hot Stuff!

- Hot food (soup, boiling water, steam, hot splashing oil, and more) can cause brutal burns on little ones. Hot oil splatters if water touches it—so be careful.

- If your kid likes to stir things on the stove, always have a grown-up hold the handle with a pot holder so it stays put. Stay within arm's reach when you're working at the stove together.

- *Keep pot handles pointed toward the back of the stove so they don't get accidentally knocked off.*

- Teach your child to never, *ever* turn on the stove or oven without an adult standing there. (And if they're too young and wild to reliably stick to the rules, pop on those kidproof oven knobs.)

- Be clear about oven safety: putting things into and taking things out of the oven is a grown-up's job only. *Always.* Period. No exceptions. (Kid's job: turning on the oven light and looking through the glass to determine whether a dish is ready to eat.)

- Keep a fire extinguisher in the kitchen and know how to use it. Baking soda can be used on small grease fires.

- Discuss safety in simple, clear terms. "We are turning on the heat now. The pan will get very hot and could burn you if you touch it." Warn kids that the stove stays hot even after the burner is turned off.

Sharp Stuff!

- Knives: teach kids that they should use only special kids' knives with the help of a grown-up sous chef. No sharp knives *ever*. Teach them that blades are very sharp and not to be touched. You know your children best, so you'll have to decide whether you think they're ready for this.

- Graters, peelers, and more: keep fingers away from the metal bumps on cheese graters and veggie-peeler blades. Canned-food lids are also sharp, and your children should know to ask an adult to help remove them. Teach kids to grate in a slow, controlled manner and to stop grating when the food gets too small to grip. A grater cut might be just a harmless bloody knuckle, but it might scare a kid right out of the kitchen, so helping kids grate and peel safely could build their confidence.

Dangerous Appliances!

- Teach your children to never turn on a blender or food processor without grown-up supervision. Only adults should put food in and out of the blender or food processor. We leave these appliances unplugged when we aren't using them.

Keep It Clean!

- Everyone washes hands before cooking. The CDC recommends singing "Happy Birthday" twice while you lather your hands with warm water and soap. Then rinse clean and pat dry.

- Everyone washes hands after handling raw meat or eggs. Scrub utensils and cutting boards after they've touched raw meat. Do not put cooked meat on the same plate where it sat raw.

- Wash all fruits and vegetables in cold running water. No soap. Scrub firm produce, like potatoes, with a brush.

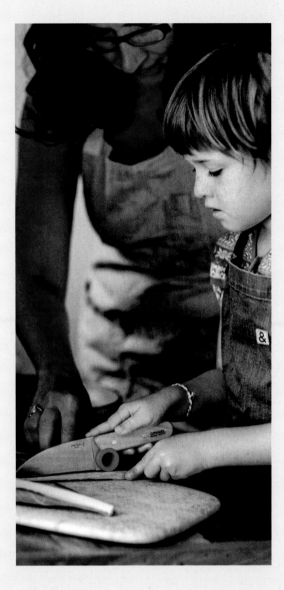

Family Kitchen Tools: Essentials

A POWERFUL BLENDER: A Vitamix will make cooking with kids much more fun. Make fresh nut milk, puree whole raw carrots, or blend smoothies—these blenders are expensive, but they last forever, and nothing beats them. Refurbished Vitamix blenders are available for a lot less, and they're just as good. Cheaper brands (like Ninja) are also effective, but make sure you check the directions before pouring hot soup or nuts into them.

MINI (THREE- TO FOUR-CUP) FOOD PROCESSOR: It's much easier to use this tiny food processor instead of a big old blender when you're making small batches of salad dressing, hummus, nut butters, or other sauces.

RICE COOKER: What did we do before this thing? Turn it on, add rice and water, forget about it.

A FEW GOOD POTS: We like enameled cast iron because it cooks evenly and is easy to clean. Le Creuset is the gold standard, but there are now many more reasonably priced imitators on the market. We're soup people so we like to use an eight-quart stockpot to make a week's worth of soup. That's pretty huge. We also keep a five-quart enameled cast-iron soup pot with a lid, which makes a perfect vessel for homemade chai and other brews. A one-and-a-half-quart saucepan with a lid works well for everything from sauces to oatmeal.

A FEW CAST-IRON FRYING PANS: Cast-iron pans distribute heat evenly, and they last forever—they're the best. They're indestructible—our kids test this daily. A ten-inch, an eight-inch, and a six-inch pan should do the trick. We also use a mini kid-size pan (three and a half inches).

MASON JARS WITH LIDS (FOUR OUNCES, EIGHT OUNCES, AND SIXTEEN OUNCES): We love these for preparing, preserving, storing, and serving food. We put yogurt parfaits in them and stuff them with salads when we go on picnics.

LARGE STAINLESS STEEL MIXING BOWLS: Whether you want to mix stuff up, serve stuff at the table, or beat the bowls like a drum, these are a staple.

STEAMER BASKET INSERT: Some of the recipes in this book require a steamer. They're supercheap, and we use ours several times a week.

Family Table Essentials

Here are some things that make our family meals more beautiful and kid friendly.

TINY TASTING BOWLS: Tiny soy sauce dipping bowls, wee ceramic prep bowls, and ramekins don't have to be fancy. We find that having a supply of these little bowls inspires our kids to eat adventurously. Little ones can be easily overwhelmed by large servings of unfamiliar foods, so we like to serve new foods in mini tasting bowls. Zero pressure. The difference between seeing four peas in a miniature soy sauce dish and a mountain of peas on an adult-size dinner plate can make all the difference for hesitant young eaters. Tiny dipping bowls like those used for soy sauce come in all shapes, colors, and materials. Espresso cups (formally known as demitasses) and shot glasses are also perfect for kid-size servings. We find that offering new foods to kids in tiny servings is key to success (and less wasteful), and we're always ready to give seconds or thirds to anyone who wants more.

KID-SIZE DRINKING CUPS (GLASS OR STAINLESS STEEL): There are plenty of kid-friendly ways to hold liquids. We prefer glass, ceramic, or stainless steel instead of plastic.

CHILD-SIZE PITCHER: Repurpose an old creamer or find a tiny ceramic or glass pitcher. Our kids really like having their own pitcher for serving themselves drinks.

SMALL WOODEN, CERAMIC, AND/OR STAINLESS STEEL BOWLS: We use these for serving kid-size portions of soup and salad.

SMALL STAINLESS FLATWARE: People are always trying to pawn off plastic utensils on kids, but kid-size stainless steel utensils last forever *and* they're dishwasher safe.

PLACE MATS: When we went to Japan for a science-fiction TV-show fan convention in 2017, the fans gave us gifts that were so beautifully wrapped we didn't even want to unwrap them. The gifts were covered in printed lightweight fabrics. We kept the fabric pieces and made them into place mats and napkins. They make dinner look fancy, and they make cleanup fast.

WOODEN PLATES WITH DIVIDERS: It's not uncommon for young kids to flip out if their various foods touch one another on the plate. These basic plates allow us to serve a few different things on one dish while keeping each item separate. The feel of wood is wonderful, but there is a downside: they can't be put in the dishwasher.

STAINLESS SPREADING KNIVES: Little cheese spreaders are perfect for little hands. We often serve dips in tiny prep dishes for kids, and they love spreading their own hummus or yogurt around.

CONDIMENT SETUP: We set up a condiment tray with kid-size containers that we bring out for every meal. Our condiment tray includes butter with a mini spreader; a bowl of pinchable sea salt; balsamic vinegar, olive oil, and soy sauce or Tamari (gluten-free soy sauce); a block of Parmesan cheese; and a mini Microplane for making Parm snow. Our kids are welcome to use any condiment on the tray on any food (yes, any food!) on their plates. Maison is a hardcore soy sauce devotee. Does she spritz it on her pasta and peas? Sure. Does her unorthodox use of it make many adults cringe? Most definitely. Ketchup was becoming too much of a go-to in our house, so we pulled it from our regular condiment tray and made a ketchup rule—it's just for hot dogs, burgers, and fries. We also make available mayonnaise and mustard (classic yellow, Dijon, and spicy brown).

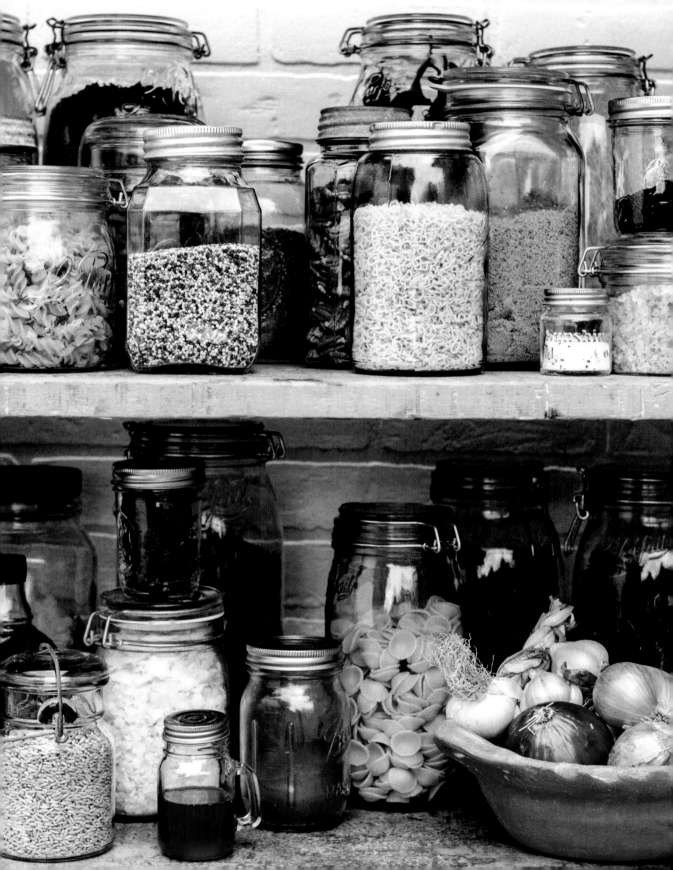

CHAPTER 4

THE NEW KID-FRIENDLY PANTRY

HERE'S A LIST of everything you need for an adventure-style pantry makeover, including staple ingredients that invite creative application. Bring on a smorgasbord of whole foods—the chunky, crunchy bites; the salty things; and the chewy sweet morsels.

We normally keep fresh, organic, minimally processed foods in our refrigerator and pantry. When work lets up, we'll even do homesteading projects like canning blackberry jam. But we know that sometimes our family is too busy and burned out to make a meal from scratch, so we also keep some canned, dried, and frozen foods on hand (like canned refried beans and frozen peas). This is, after all, the twenty-first century. Every one of us—especially parents, since we're some of the most exhausted people on the planet—needs convenient foods sometimes.

Finally, as you're building your unique family pantry, remember that organized shelves invite spontaneous cooking projects because they make it easy to see what's on hand. We like to use large glass jars for storing grains, oats, beans, nuts, and dried fruit so we can see all those dazzling textures and colors. Here are our favorite staples from our kid-friendly adventure pantry.

The Basics: Fridge

BUTTER: This creamy dairy goodness is the best thing since sliced bread. No, that's not right—it's the best thing *on* sliced bread. We have cases of our homemade jams just waiting to be devoured, and it would be a crime not to butter our toast before slathering on the homemade jam. There are certain things like peas that taste better with butter, too. But if you're not into butter, coconut oil is a good substitute. There's also ghee, a form of butter traditionally used in Asian cooking, which is made from cow's milk but is lower in lactose than butter.

CHEESE: We like cheese for a few reasons: (1) it's why cows were invented; (2) it's delicious; (3) kids love grating, and cheese loves to be grated; (4) there are a huge variety of cheeses, and allowing kids to taste and compare them gives them a chance to expand their palates.

ON SEASONAL, LOCAL, AND ORGANIC PRODUCE

Organics

We buy organic whenever possible. We realize we're lucky, because organic food isn't cheap and can be cost-prohibitive for many families. If your family can spring for *some* organic produce, check out the Clean 15 and Dirty Dozen annual lists to see which fruits and vegetables contain the most pesticide residue before deciding where to invest your organic dollars. These lists are helpful because they let you know which organic produce might be worth shelling out an extra buck for and which may not be. For example, there are lots of pesticides on conventionally grown spinach but barely any on conventionally grown avocados, so you could save a buck by skipping the organic avocado and spend it on organic spinach instead.

Seasonal

Have you ever eaten a grocery-store tomato in January? That pallid, hard, flavorless bite pales when compared with a ripe summer tomato. That's why we've experimented with growing tomatoes, kale, and salad greens in our garden. Our kids love harvesting straight from the plant, and there's nothing like a tomato pulled right off the vine—sliced, salted, and dipped in olive oil. But as much as we dream about growing all our own food, it's just not something we can manage in real life. We do relish eating with the seasons so we try to find in-season veggies at the store or farmers' market. We've also planted herbs like sage and rosemary, which are so hearty they could pretty much survive in a vacant parking lot.

Orange cheese often contains artificial colors, stabilizers, and preservatives. Plus, it tends to be code for "kids' menu" and "processed food," and we don't want our kids to think that orange cheese is the only edible cheese, so we just don't stock it at home. If kids eat orange cheese out in the world, no biggie. There's so much to explore in the cheese world. We stock blocks (so the kids can grate them) of Parmesan, mild Cheddar, provolone, and a rotation of other cheeses for the kids to try. We don't stock preshredded cheese, as it contains anticaking chemicals, and it doesn't melt as nicely. Our kids are still hesitant about the bold flavors of pungent cheeses, but bite by bite, they're discovering the miraculous phenomenon of cheese.

FRESH HERBS: Fresh herbs have pride of place in our house. We grow a few basic herbs like rosemary, chives, and sage. We also love walking around looking for fresh herbs growing in our 'hood. Do not report us, but we will steal a couple of sprigs if we think they won't be missed. To keep them fresh longer, snip the stems and put them in a glass of water in the fridge.

FROZEN FRUIT AND VEGGIES: Our favorite frozen fruits include blueberries, mangoes, pineapple, strawberries, and raspberries. Our favorite frozen veggies include peas, corn, edamame (both shelled and in the shell), carrots, and spinach. We throw frozen fruits and frozen spinach in smoothies. We use frozen peas, corn, and carrots when we want to make easy fried rice and shepherd's pie. Edamame is one of our favorite easy snacks.

LEMONS AND LIMES: We use freshly squeezed lemon or lime juice daily. There are so many foods that are brought to life by a little sour squirt, and juicing citrus is a perfect project for foodies in training.

The Basics: Pantry

AROMATICS: Fresh onions, garlic, and shallots don't need to be refrigerated, so we keep them in a bowl on the counter.

CANNED AND JARRED GOODS: We keep marinara sauce (find one with no added sugar), canned tomatoes, tomato paste, vegetable broth, and chicken broth on our shelves, along with canned legumes such as garbanzo beans, pinto beans, black beans, and refried beans. They're convenient, and opening a can is a wicked good time for a kid.

COLD-PRESSED EXTRA-VIRGIN OLIVE OIL AND BALSAMIC VINEGAR: West pours balsamic vinegar on everything from raw spinach to pasta. He drank it from the bottle once, then complained about his sore tongue. If your child is a fan of vinegary flavors, there are plenty of vinegars to explore—in addition to balsamic, we keep apple cider and white wine vinegars in the cupboard. We use a lot of cold-pressed extra-virgin olive oil. Other oils that we keep on hand for sautéing and frying include peanut, sesame, safflower, canola, and coconut. Olive and canola have relatively high smoke points, so they work well for sautéing over medium-high heat. Oils with higher smoke points (such as coconut, safflower, corn, peanut, and sesame) are ideal for high-heat frying and stir-frying.

DRIED BEANS: We keep dried beans (store-bought) in the pantry. Some of our favorites include garbanzo beans, lentils, mung beans, split peas, pinto beans, and black beans.

DRIED HERBS AND SPICES: Our inventory includes vanilla beans, whole nutmeg (which is fun to grate with a Microplane or fine grater), cinnamon sticks and ground cinnamon, cardamom pods, whole cloves, cumin, basil, turmeric,

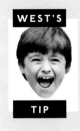

WEST'S TIP

Check out the stickers on your fruit. Where did your apples come from? Can you map how many miles that apple has traveled to get to you? Do you think it took boats or planes or trains to get to you?

oregano, and paprika. Younger kids might have a blast opening jarred herbs and spices and sniffing them. We let West and Maison use small amounts of herbs and spices that have been in the cabinet for a very long time when they make their "concoctions"—watching herbs get poured into an inedible paste isn't easy; we tell ourselves that our kids are doing important kid work by getting to know the look and smell of various seasonings. This familiarity will, we hope, make them less likely to freak out when confronted with a particle of cumin on a dinner plate. Even if it means they're just having fun in the kitchen, that's a win, too.

DRIED FRUITS: We like to keep a supply of dried fruit from the bulk-foods section of the market around. Did you know that dried fruit often contains added preservatives and sweeteners, like corn syrup? Dried fruit is supersweet—there's no need to get the kind with added sugar. Choose unsweetened sulfur-free dried fruit: it doesn't have the same vivid color, but it also doesn't have added chemical preservatives. Our favorite dried fruits are apricots, dates, raisins, mangoes, blueberries, and pineapple.

FLOUR: All-purpose flour is the workhorse of the pantry. It's good for bread, pizza dough, pie crust, muffins, cakes, biscuits, waffles, pancakes, imitation Play-Doh, papier-mâché, and just throwing at your children. We use the unbleached variety because it goes through less chemical processing than bleached flour.

GRAINS: Rice (we like the brown, jasmine, wild, and forbidden varieties), cornmeal, couscous, giant (or Israeli) couscous, millet, oats, and quinoa. We keep our grains in glass jars because it's easy to see what we have.

NUTS AND SEEDS OF ALL KINDS: Our favorites include chia, flax, pumpkin, sesame, and poppy seeds along with almonds, cashews, hazelnuts, pecans, pine nuts, pistachios, peanuts, and walnuts. Nuts can be stored in the pantry for up to three months, but they last longer in the fridge. We consume nuts and seeds enthusiastically, so we don't usually have them hanging around the pantry for long.

NUT BUTTERS: We also like to keep nut butters on hand. Most peanut butters these days contain added sugar and chemicals, so look for old-school peanut butter with two ingredients only: peanuts and salt. It'll have oil on top, and you'll have to stir it when you first crack it open, which is messy and inconvenient, but it's much more healthful and tastier, so it's worth it. We also love almond butter.

PASTA: We like to stock a bunch of different shapes and types of pasta. Semolina (wheat) pasta is the traditional Italian variety. We also stock pasta made from brown rice and quinoa to mix it up.

SALT: It's a well-kept secret that salt is the key to delicious meals. We keep a big Diamond Crystal salt container next to the stove. That's what we throw in when we're boiling water for pasta. We recently discovered how many finishing-salt options are out there . . . pink Himalayan, black smoked, truffle. We have fallen in love with the flaky crystals of Maldon sea salt. It's a finishing salt that isn't intended for cooking. Be warned: this is an embarrassingly expensive luxury salt, so treat it like gold and sprinkle it on your food just before serving. It's fun to explore various salts—smoky black salt on popcorn? In our family, we have two salt fiends: Misha and Maison. Misha likes things quite salty, and Maison will treat salt like a food and eat it straight out of the box. (Should we be worried?)

> *For children to eat well, food has to be tasty and well prepared. To be tasty and well prepared, food has to contain fat. . . . Fat with food helps it to taste good and gives it a slippery quality that makes it easier for a young child to chew and swallow. . . . Fat enhances food flavor; sugar disguises it.*
>
> —ELLYN SATTER,
> therapist and international
> authority on feeding children

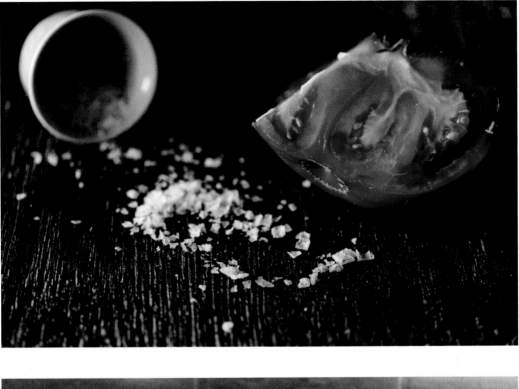

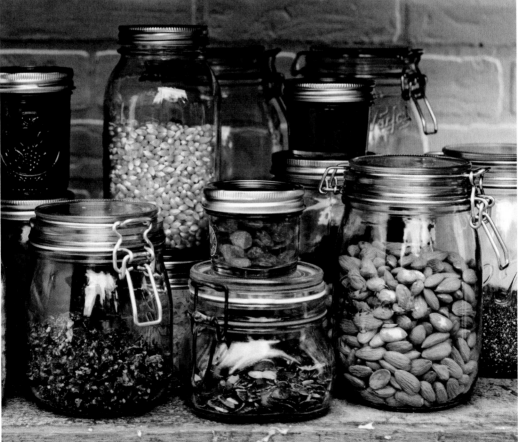

FOODS

WE DON'T KEEP AT HOME

While we indulge in the occasional potato chip and hot dog, we decided not to keep these kid staples at home. We noticed that when we kept foods like frozen pizza and hot dogs at home, we were just too tempted to serve them nightly as the go-to kids' dinner. So we made a bold decision—we stopped stocking them. We aren't purists—these foods aren't taboo for us, they're just foods that we don't usually keep around.

More foods we don't stock at home because they contain preservatives, added sugars, and other ingredients we prefer not to rely on: potato chips, Goldfish, chocolate milk, fruit juice, soda, granola bars, "protein" bars, sweetened dried fruit, prepackaged fruit snacks, sweet cold breakfast cereals, boxed mac 'n' cheese, flavored yogurt, and processed cheeses like Kraft Singles.

As a rule, we avoid commercially packaged foods with too many hard-to-pronounce ingredients, and we try not to be fooled by supposedly good-for-you foods, like sweetened banana chips and dried cranberries, which are usually coated in corn syrup or other forms of sugar. This isn't about restriction or deprivation. Sometimes a family really *needs* to top a pizza with jelly beans. We're all for it. But we found that by stocking food we want our family to eat, we eliminated some not-so-fun food-related negotiations at home and lessened our own temptation to fall into the easy kid-menu rut.

After all, one area of life that parents *can* control is what food comes into the home. Instead of nagging kids about eating this or that, we find it's easier to just stock the whole foods we want them to eat. We relish that prerogative.

If you've been serving the standard kids'-food diet at home and you're thinking about shifting toward more whole foods, consider a bold move: start by letting your boxed mac 'n' cheese supply dwindle. It's too easy to get overwhelmed by all the health-related shoulds and shouldn'ts, but . . . when *was* the last time you read the ingredients list on a box of mac 'n' cheese? Did you know that most kinds of boxed mac 'n' cheese, including brands marketed as healthy, use artificial color, preservatives, and stabilizers? Just because a food is marketed as "natural" doesn't mean it's good for you. Check the ingredients. You might not be able to pronounce many items on the list. If that feels too overwhelming, there's a simpler option. Buy items with an ingredient list of one. Broccoli is made from broccoli.

SWEETENERS: Molasses, pure maple syrup (we like *all* real maple syrups—our favorite is grade B because it's thicker, darker, and more mapley in flavor than grade A), stevia powder or liquid (a glycemic index of zero), honey (unsafe for kids under the age of one), brown sugar, and white sugar.

Shopping with Kids

Every parent knows that grocery shopping with kids can be fun—or it can be a journey into the depths of hell. The upside: it allows kids to see an entire universe of foods. Sometimes we do a grocery store "scavenger hunt." We'll say, "Quick, West, grab five bananas. Maison, find two green veggies to put in our cart." On a good day, it's fun. On a not-so-good day, we'll find ourselves in a textbook food-related power struggle. The food industry's marketing teams aren't dummies. They make sure the junkiest foods—from sugary cereals to candy bars—are perfectly positioned on shelves at a child's eye level. If you've ever watched *Cooking Fast & Fresh with West*, you'll see what gems will end up in your cart when you turn a two-year-old loose in a grocery store. At first, we found it hilarious to let West roam through the store and choose whatever his toddler heart desired . . . then it was not so funny. (We know; we were asking for it.) He'd bite into a raw red cabbage, then erupt into a full-blown tantrum when we refused to buy ten (yes, ten) one-pound bags of Starbursts (and yes, he needed *all* of them, immediately). To avoid the M&M's Meltdowns™, we had to set out firm rules in advance of every trip. And yes, we have to repeat them. Every. Single. Trip. We learned that we needed to be in charge of which foods came home with us—and setting up clear shopping parameters in advance makes for a smoother shopping experience for everyone.

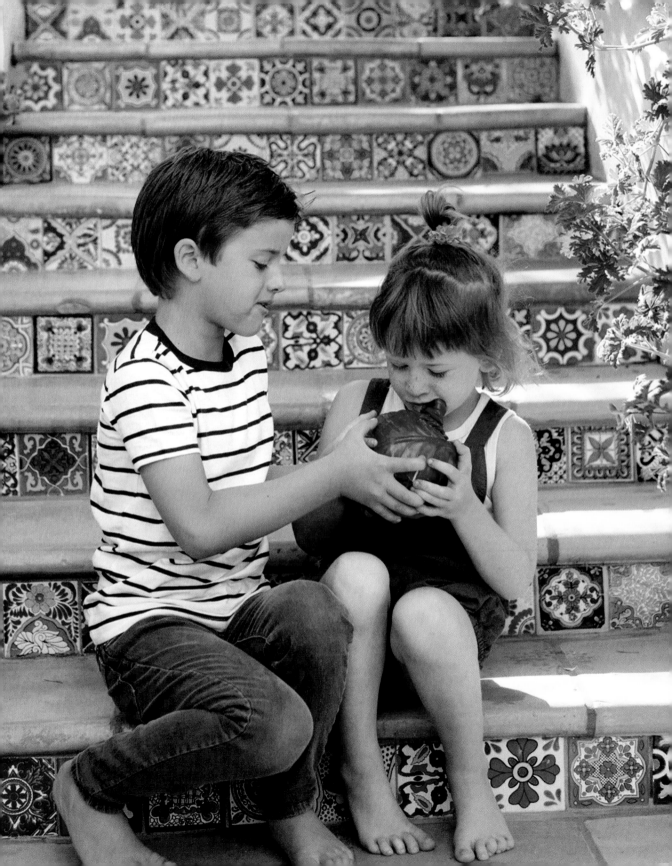

CHAPTER 5

HOW TO USE THIS BOOK

THERE ARE TWO kinds of people in the world—those who follow recipes religiously and the rest of us. We provide measurements and instructions in this cookbook, but we have a moral responsibility to inform you that these recipes are meant to be improvised upon. They're meant to bring the family together—and if that means you follow every instruction together gleefully, go for it. If it means you veer wildly from the recipe, we encourage that, too. As long as your family is having fun and getting inspired about food together, you're using this book as it was meant to be used.

MEASUREMENTS: We give specific measurements in our recipes. These amounts are meant only as a guide. Still, the recipes in this book are resilient and forgiving. Don't worry about getting them exactly right. Why use measuring spoons when you can use your hands? Put in a fistful of this. A pinch of that. A drizzle . . . a dab . . . a dollop.

SUBSTITUTIONS: Here's what we say if you don't have an ingredient: substitute, by all means. Can't find yogurt? Try sour cream. Don't have Cheddar but you've got Parmesan? Go for it. You get the idea. Omissions and additions to the recipes are welcome according to your family's likes, dislikes, and whims. You have our full permission to let your kids add, substitute, or swap out. Also, your creations don't need to look like our creations. Yours will have their own unique appearance.

NOTE ON INGREDIENTS: When we call for eggs, we mean large eggs. You only have small eggs laid by your neighbor's pet chicken? Okay—the meal will not be ruined if you use those. When we call for bread, any sliced bread will do. We happen to be fans of seedy wholegrain bread (especially the Ezekiel brand) and freshly baked bread from our local bakery. When we call for butter, we mean salted butter because we're a salt-loving family. If you aren't keen on salt, or if you prefer to control the salt content carefully, use unsalted butter, by all means. When we call for milk, any milk will do. Sometimes we use organic whole milk; other times we use almond milk.

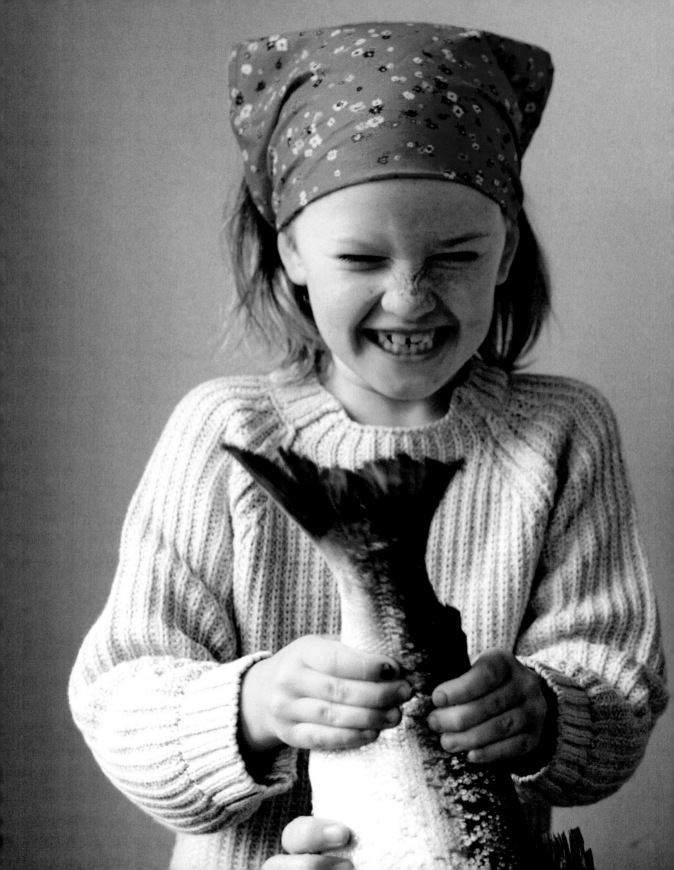

PART II

ADVENTUROUS RECIPES

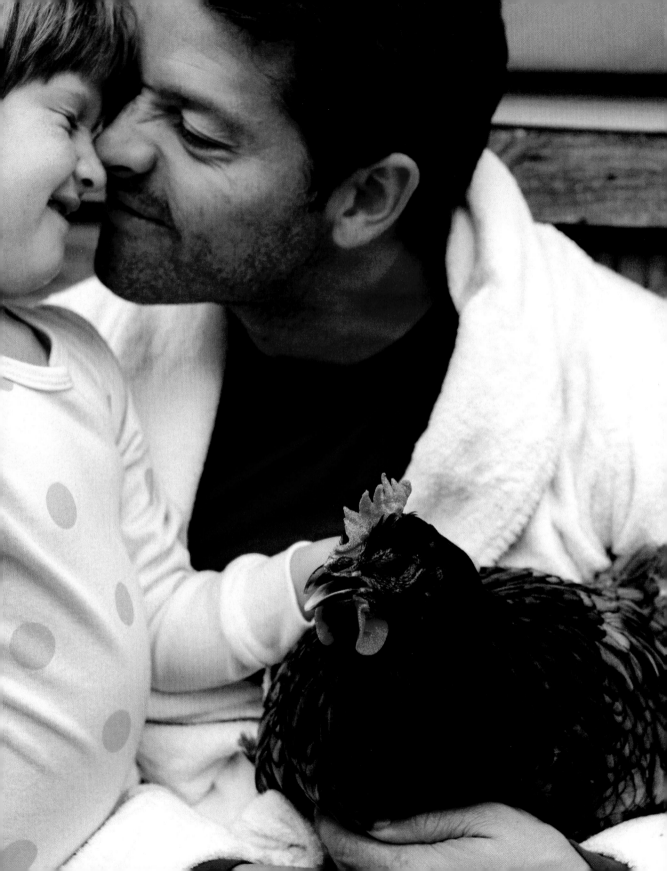

THE
BREAKFAST CLUB

f you've ever had to pry a box of Cocoa Puffs from a toddler's hands, you understand how deep the love is between kids and sugary cereals. Of *course* kids go cuckoo for Cocoa Puffs. Cereal manufacturers employ teams of food scientists devoted to concocting just the right chemical brew to give cereal the perfect texture, sweetness, look, and "mouth feel." What kid wouldn't be wooed by this irresistible laboratory-perfected breakfast?

One of the problems with sugar-coated cereals and their advertising is that they teach kids that food has to be candylike to be edible, and they mask the yummy (albeit subtler) taste of real grains. If kids get too used to the flavor and texture of these highly processed foods, they may grow to reject steel-cut oats.

When we stocked store-bought granola and other boxed breakfast cereals in our home, we initially thought they were healthful, but when we checked the ingredients, we found that many faux-healthful cereals branded as "natural" are packed with sugar and preservatives. Moreover, our kids seemed to get addicted to it. Soon they wanted cold cereal every day for breakfast, lunch, dinner, and an after-dinner snack. Eventually we phased it out of our pantry. Now we only stock unsweetened hippie cereal. This way, we have cereal when we need a superfast breakfast, but our kids won't obsess over it.

MISHA SAYS: My grandfather managed the Domino sugar factory in New York City, and it was there that he developed what every American can agree was a life-changing invention: brownulated sugar—"The brown sugar that pours!" Hence my grandparents heralded sugar as "pure energy!" This meant that when my brother and I stayed at their house, we could—and did—eat nearly infinite amounts of the stuff. At breakfast, we would pour so much sugar on our corn-flakes that our spoons would stand upright in the milk.

Now, we don't want to mislead anyone here. We understand the real miracle that cold cereal is—it generates time for parents. It's a lightning-fast breakfast that kids can make on their own, thereby buying parents an extra thirteen seconds to shower, brush their teeth, or sleep. This can be a lifesaver if your family's morning routine feels like a fire drill, which is often the case in our household. "No, I'm *not* going to wear that!!" "Where's my sock?" "Why are you starting a puzzle *now*? We're going to be late for school—*again!*"

Would it be lovely to have an extra hour in the morning to make creative breakfasts and eat a civilized meal together? Indeed. That's probably not in the cards for most of us. But is cold cereal the only option?

Maybe not.

We've included our family's favorite breakfasts in this chapter—many are quick enough for rushed weekday mornings, and they all invite kid improvisation, participation, and innovation—when there's time.

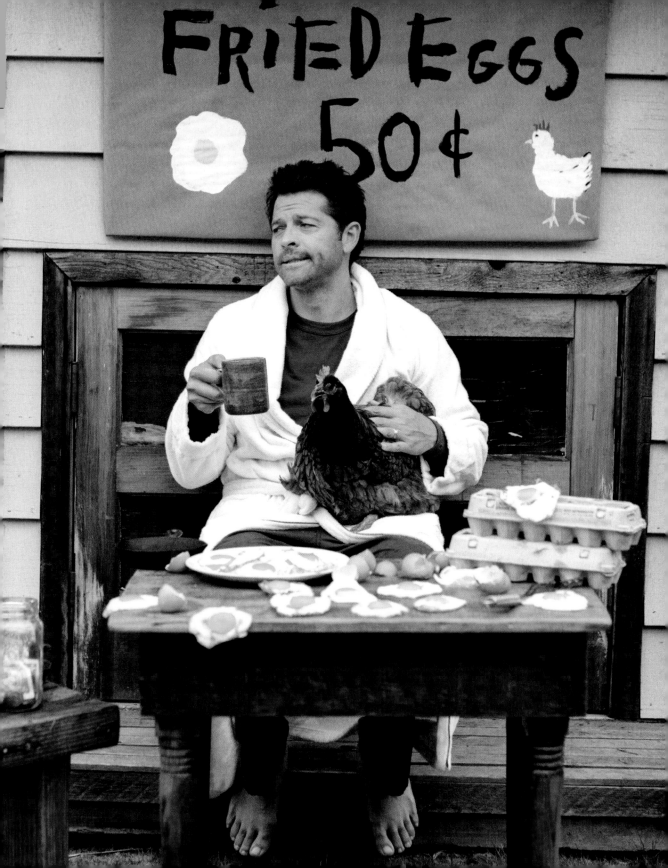

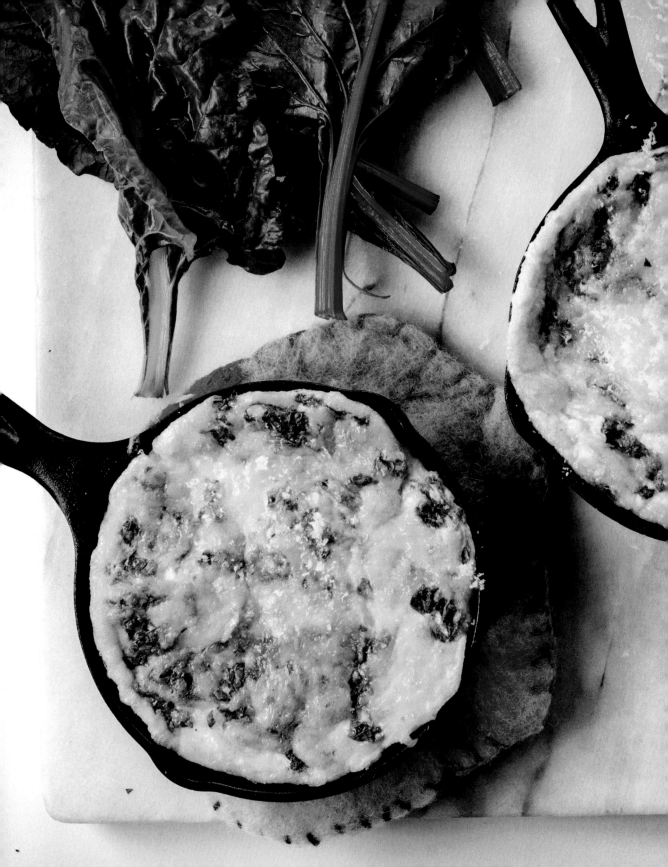

CONFETTI FRITTATA

SERVES 4 TO 6

1 leaf Swiss or rainbow chard (Yes, just one leaf—the goal here is to introduce the visual of leafy green specks without altering the flavor or texture.)

6 eggs

1 cup milk

Sea salt to taste

2 tablespoons butter

¾ cup grated mild Cheddar cheese

¾ cup grated Swiss cheese or Gruyère cheese

When Misha was a kid and money was really tight one winter, his family lived in a tent in the woods. Without a refrigerator, they stored food in a picnic cooler with ice. If they didn't eat perishables quickly, they'd spoil. When dairy products were on the verge of going bad, Misha's mom would make a quiche in a cast-iron pan over the campfire. Misha loved it. The first time we served quiche to our kids, however, they were not impressed. West eyed it suspiciously and barely mustered the courage to poke it with his fork. "What *is* it? What are those green things?" No amount of cajoling would persuade him to taste it. So we enlisted him to help us invent a simple, crustless version (aka a frittata). After seeing every ingredient that went into it, he was willing to take a bite, albeit cautiously. "It's actually pretty good," he reported. One of the wonders of frittatas is that they work with almost any combo of veggies, and now that frittatas are part of our family's repertoire, we use them to explore new veggie varieties. It can be a super simple affair, or it can be an improvisational playground for the whole family. This version uses a single leaf of chard (snipped into "confetti") to ease kids into relishing green specks.

Preheat the oven to 350°F.

Kid's job! Wash and dry the chard. Hold the stem at the bottom, like a handle, in one hand. Use your other hand to tear the leaf away from the stem in one swoop. Set aside the stem or use it for a duel. Using child scissors, snip off tiny pieces of the leaf to make teeny green confetti. Set aside.

Combine the eggs, milk, and salt in a medium mixing bowl and whisk until well mixed.

Melt the butter in a medium-size pan (preferably cast iron) over medium heat. Swirl the butter so it coats all sides of the pan. Once the pan is evenly coated, pour the excess melted butter into the whisked eggs and give them a stir. Set aside.

continued

Add the chard confetti to the pan and stir until just wilted. If there's water in the pan after sautéing the greens, press the greens into the pan with a spatula and tip the pan to pour out the excess into the sink.

Pour the egg mixture into the pan. Top one side of the pan with Cheddar and the other with Swiss or Gruyère. Pop the pan in the oven and bake for 20 minutes. Stick a toothpick in the middle: if it comes out mostly clean, it's ready.

Let the frittata cool for a few minutes, then slice into wedges and serve.

EGGS À LA INSECTS, ANYONE?

Consider this thought experiment, parents. When you're feeling frustrated as all heck by your child's resistance to consuming a new food (such as a frittata), imagine putting a mystery meat in your mouth that tastes and feels like nothing you've ever eaten before. You have no idea what it is or how it's been prepared. How hard is it for you to force yourself to swallow it? Now think of a food that gives you the heebie-jeebies—something you're incapable of tasting because the thought of it makes you shudder.

For young children, the shudder-inducing food could be scrambled eggs or carrots. Kids often find it hard to cope with a new food—especially when it's served out of context and they have no idea where it came from or how it was prepared.

Remember that it can take any of us (even adults) a while to get comfortable with a new food. Studies show that it can take young kids up to fifteen exposures to a food before they're willing to taste it. There's a chance your kid might taste something new sooner if they've been involved in the cooking process, know a little bit about the food, and have had the chance to smell the food and play with it. Children's sensory systems need time and exposure to adapt to the smell, sight, touch, taste, and even the sound of a new food before they're ready to eat it. So when a kid says, "I don't like that," often what they really mean is: "I'm not ready for that" or "That's too challenging to eat right now."

EGG AND CHEESE CUPCAKES

MAKES 6 CUPCAKES

Butter for greasing

6 slices bread

1¼ cups grated Parmesan, Cheddar, or Jack cheese, divided

6 eggs

Pinch of sea salt

Cupcakes are the perfect food—mostly because they fit in little hands. A savory twist on the classic—these eggy, protein-packed "cupcakes" make a perfect on-the-go breakfast.

Preheat the oven to 375°F. Butter a 6-cup muffin tin.

Kid's job! Press the rim of a sturdy drinking glass into a slice of bread to make a round cutout. Using your glass, stamp out six rounds of bread. Grab the crusty bread scraps and rip 'em up into nickel-size pieces. Put those ripped bread bits in a pile.

Distribute 1 cup of grated cheese evenly among the muffin cups—the cheese will crisp and form a crust on the bottom while baking. Press one bread round firmly into the bottom of each cup, on top of the layer of cheese.

Kid's job! Give the eggs and salt a good whisking in a large Pyrex measuring cup (or any large cup or bowl with a pour spout). Pour the eggs into each muffin cup. Go slowly . . . can you fill each cup almost to the top without spilling over?

Top each cup with the reserved bread scraps, sprinkle the remaining ¼ cup cheese over the top, and bake for 25 minutes. Let cool for a few minutes before serving.

KIDS ▶ GRATE CHEESE SIDEWAYS

Teach your parents this grating trick. Instead of standing the box grater up, lay it on its side on top of a cutting board, big holes facing up. (When grating, remember to keep your fingers away from the little blades and only grate big pieces of food. The sideways grate makes nicking your fingers less likely—plus, anything is more fun when you do it sideways.) Grab a big block of Parmesan cheese with the hand you write with. Hold the grater handle with the other hand to keep it from slipping and sliding. Now grate, grate, grate your cheese horizontally on top of the sideways grater until you have a mini cheese mountain inside your grater.

THE PIRATE'S EYE
(AKA THE BIRD IN THE NEST)

SERVES 2

2 slices bread

1 to 2 tablespoons butter

2 eggs

Sea salt to taste

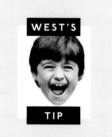

WEST'S TIP

Try my favorite pirate joke (it's funnier when you use a pirate accent):

Q: Why does it take pirates so long to learn the alphabet?

A: Because they can spend years at c.

Misha could eat eggs every morning. Share a new egg-poaching tip and he's rapt. In our family, we love this classic eggy breakfast because our kids can practically make it by themselves. West prefers only egg whites, and he likes them fried into a super-crispy, nearly burned state that would make most egg snobs shudder. We let him cook this exactly the way he likes it. We have to stand right next to him—it does involve a hot stove—but it's still a perfect rushed morning breakfast since it takes about four minutes to make. Sometimes we take it to go and eat it on the way to school.

Kid's job! Make a 2-inch-ish hole in the center of each slice of bread. Use child scissors to cut the bread, or press the rim of a drinking glass into the bread to make the hole. Or tear out a hole with your bare hands while snarling like Captain Sparrow.

Melt the butter in a small pan over medium heat. Once it's starting to bubble, put one slice of the holey bread in the pan. Sear it for about 1 to 2 minutes, or until nicely browned, then flip it. Crack an egg into the hole in the bread, then sprinkle with salt. Cover the pan and cook for about 3 minutes, then uncover and, using a spatula, transfer the egg-in-a-hole to a plate. Repeat with the second slice of bread and egg.

If your kids like eggs cooked hard, once you turn off the heat, you can leave the lid on the pan and let it sit for an additional minute or two. The residual heat will cook the egg a bit more without charring the bread.

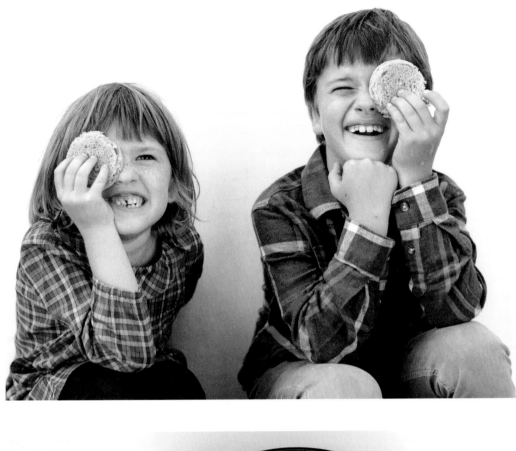

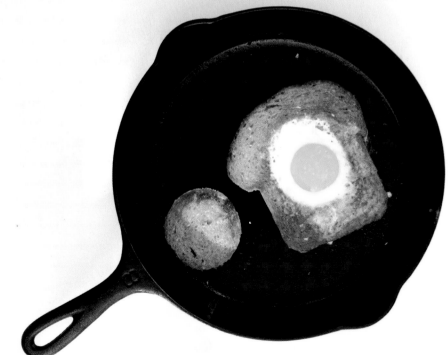

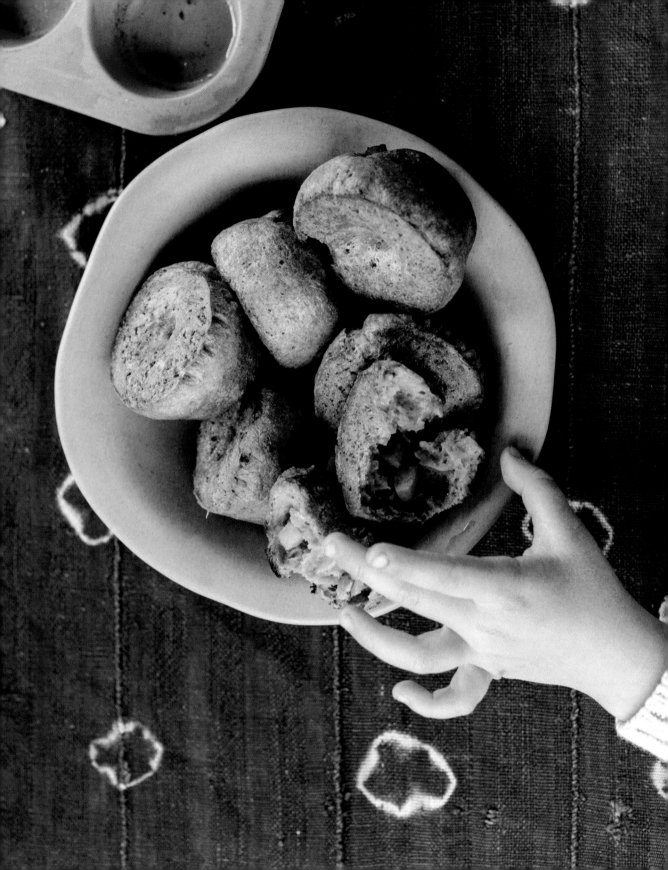

GREEN EGGS AND HAM POPOVERS

MAKES 12 POPOVERS

5 tablespoons melted butter

4 eggs

1½ cups milk

¼ cup firmly packed baby spinach

Pinch of sea salt

1½ cups all-purpose flour

½ cup chopped cooked ham

The first book West ever read aloud to us was Dr. Seuss's *Green Eggs and Ham*. Inspired by this famous breakfast tale, we invented our own green eggs and ham recipe. It gives kids a chance to eat a spinach-green breakfast with an easy-to-love bready texture. Maison says, "I do like green eggs and ham!"

Preheat the oven to 450°F. Position a rack in the lower part of the oven.

Kid's job! Put ½ teaspoon melted butter in each muffin cup of a standard 12-cup muffin tin. Brush the top of the muffin tin as well to keep the popovers from sticking to the top.

In a blender, combine the milk and the spinach. Puree until the milk turns green.

Kid's job! Throw your eggs, green milk, and salt into a large bowl. Get your whisk on. Add the flour all at once and whisk until there are no more big lumps. Stir in the remaining melted butter and the ham. Pour into a pitcher.

Divide the batter among the greased cups.

Bake for 20 minutes without opening the oven door, then reduce the heat to 350°F. Bake for 15 to 20 minutes longer, or until the popovers are nicely browned. Serve warm with a pat of butter on top.

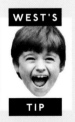

WEST'S TIP

The fun part about popovers is that they pop up while baking. Don't open the oven door while they're baking or they'll sink. Turn the oven light on and peek through the oven door.

WEST'S MONKEY BOWL

SERVES 4

2 cups rolled oats

1 to 2 tablespoons butter

One banana, sliced

½ cup pecan halves

Milk for serving

Maple syrup for serving

Even on rushed mornings, we love this hot breakfast. After all, oatmeal only takes a few minutes to cook. Here's our monkey take on this wholesome grain.

Prepare oatmeal according to package directions.

While the oatmeal is cooking, throw the butter into a hot skillet. Let it melt. Add banana slices and let them brown slightly on both sides so they caramelize. No need to be too precise.

Kid's job! Crush those pecans. What's your crushing device of choice? Mallet? Rolling pin? Mortar and pestle?

Scoop cooked oatmeal into bowls. Top with gooey banana slices, a handful of chopped pecans, a splash of milk, and a drizzle of maple syrup.

OATMEAL SUNDAE BAR

Sometimes we lay out an "oatmeal sundae" toppings bar—ramekins filled with proteiny fun toppings like raw sunflower seeds, fresh berries, chopped apples, crushed walnuts, chia seeds, and sliced almonds. Also on the table: honey and milk. Grown-ups choose which ingredients are available. Kids get to decide what they want on top.

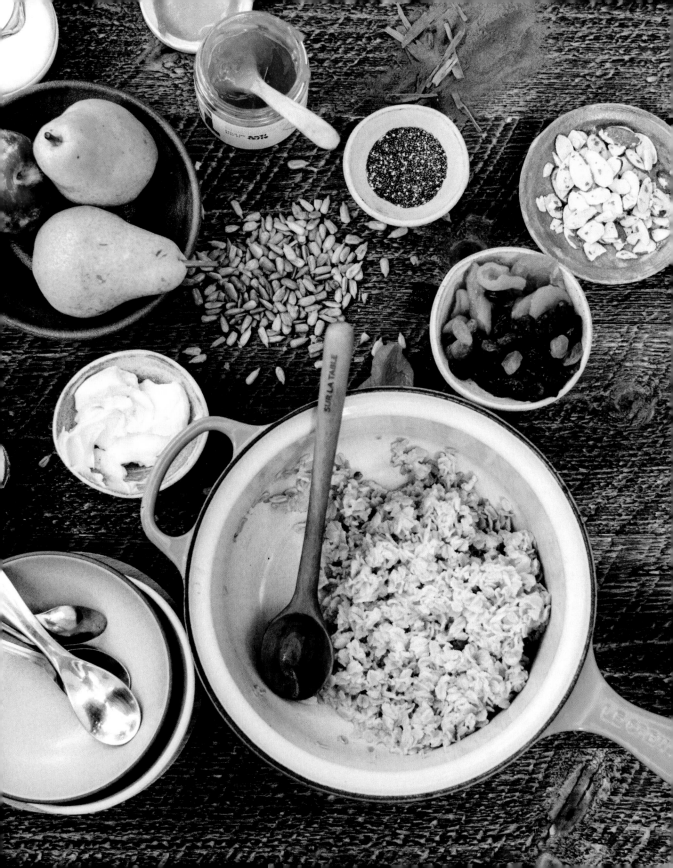

FOR-REAL, BETTER-THAN-ANY-CEREAL-YOU-COULD-BUY-AT-THE-GROCERY-STORE GRANOLA

MAKES 8 CUPS

1 cup almonds

1 cup pecans

1 cup walnuts

2½ cups rolled oats

½ cup shelled
pumpkin seeds

½ teaspoon ground
cinnamon

Pinch of sea salt

½ cup dried mango
slices, unsweetened
and preferably
unsulfured

2 egg whites

¼ cup coconut oil

¼ cup maple syrup

¼ cup honey

1 teaspoon
vanilla extract

We love making granola because kids can be involved at almost every step. Your kids can put their special stamp on it and make it their own. Here is our family's favorite recipe. We keep the sweetener light, and add egg whites for extra crunch and protein.

Preheat the oven to 350°F.

Kid's job! Smash your nuts. Put your almonds, pecans, and walnuts in a zip-lock bag. Let the extra air out. Using a rolling pin, smash those nuts into smaller pieces. If you don't have a rolling pin, you can use the bottom of a heavy pan.

Kid's job! Mix your dry stuff. Combine oats, almonds, pecans, walnuts, pumpkin seeds, cinnamon, and salt in a large bowl. Snip the mango slices into tiny pieces using child scissors and set aside.

Lightly beat the egg whites.

Melt the coconut oil, maple syrup, and honey in a small saucepan over low heat. Stir in the vanilla and egg whites. Heat until warm, then pour into the oatmeal mixture.

Kid's job! Using a wooden spoon or clean, bare hands, mix thoroughly. Spread the mixture onto two cookie sheets.

Bake for 20 to 25 minutes, stirring halfway through. Add the mango pieces and bake 3 to 5 minutes longer, or until the granola is nicely browned. Let it cool completely. Serve with plain unsweetened yogurt or milk. The granola can be stored in an airtight container for up to three weeks.

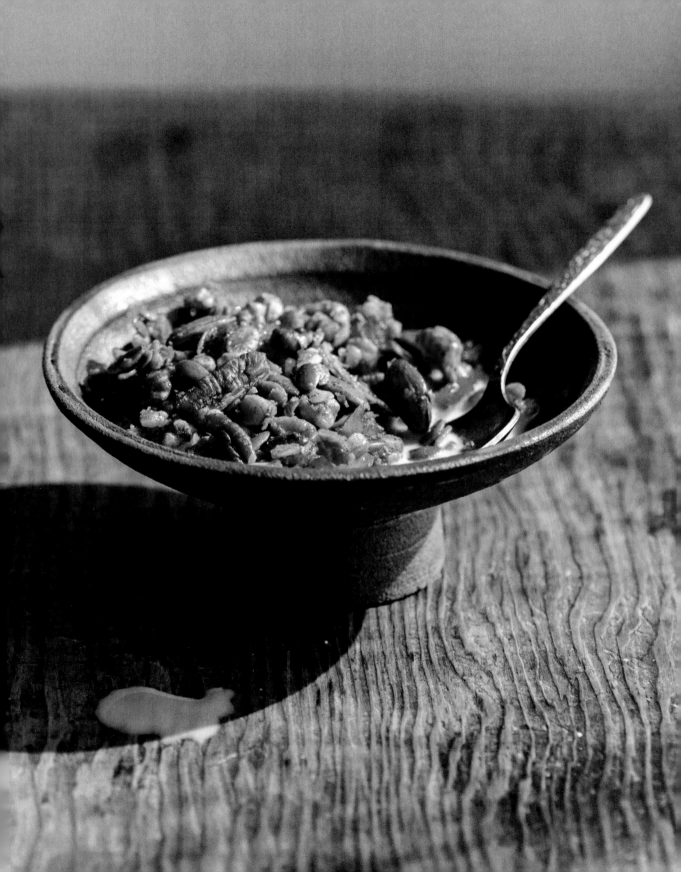

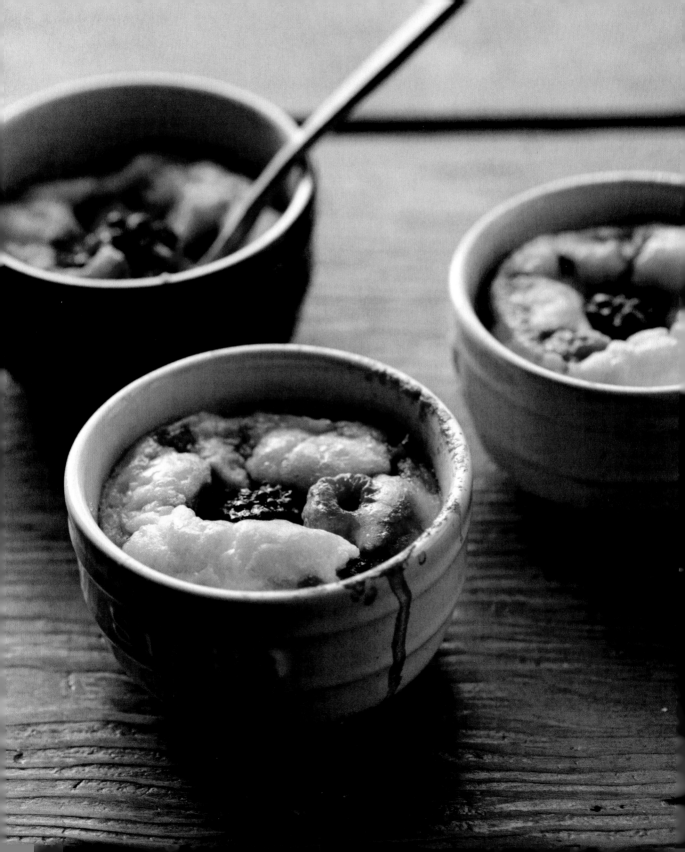

PEAR-BERRY BREAKFAST CAKE

**MAKES 6
INDIVIDUAL CAKES**

I can (15 ounces) pear halves or pear slices in unsweetened pear juice

4 tablespoons butter

4 eggs

½ cup all-purpose flour

Pinch of sea salt

1½ cups fresh raspberries or blackberries

This breakfast cake is not too sweet at all. The fruit flavors it naturally, and it's packed with eggy goodness. It's custardy and scrumptious served warm.

Preheat the oven to 375°F.

Drain the pear halves or slices, reserving the juice. Roughly chop the pears and set aside.

Melt the butter in a small saucepan over medium-low heat. When it is just melted, brush some of it on the insides of six 6-ounce ramekins. Reserve the remaining butter for the batter.

Combine the eggs, pear juice, flour, remaining melted butter, and salt in a blender or food processor. Blend until smooth—a few seconds.

Kid's job! Put some chopped pears in each of the buttered ramekins, then top each with a couple berries. Pour the batter over the fruit, distributing it evenly among the ramekins. Set the ramekins on a baking sheet.

Bake for 25 to 30 minutes.

Let cool for about 3 minutes, serve warm.

PINK YOGURT PARFAITS

MAKES 4 PARFAITS

½ cup chopped fresh strawberries

½ cup fresh raspberries

½ tablespoon honey

2 cups unsweetened plain yogurt

I cup homemade (see recipe on page 66) or store-bought granola

I tablespoon raw sunflower seeds

Instead of stocking up on those prepackaged overly sweet yogurts at the store, make your own yogurt breakfasts. These are quick and healthful, and they call for kid participation. And the layers are oh-so-pink.

Combine the strawberries, raspberries, honey, and two tablespoons of water in a blender. Blend until ultrasmooth.

Kid's job! Layer it up. Spoon a thin layer of the strawberry mixture on the bottom of four 4-ounce mason jars. Then to each jar, add a layer of about ¼ cup yogurt, a couple of tablespoons of granola, and a few sunflower seeds. Repeat layering until all ingredients are used. Do it your way.

INVENTORS' CIRCLE

What crushed seed or nut would be tasty in your yogurt parfait?

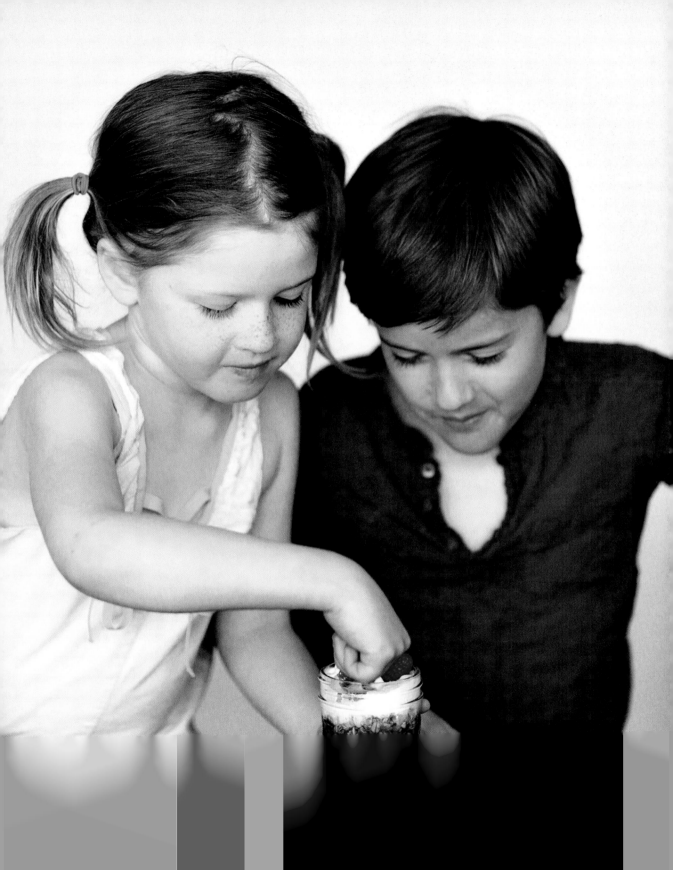

SLEEPING OATS

MAKES 4 SERVINGS

2 cups rolled oats, divided

2 cups milk, or more or less as needed, divided

2 teaspoons honey, divided

8 pinches of cinnamon

2 teaspoons vanilla extract, divided

32 raisins

Every parent knows the real reason cold cereal exists . . . so your kids can serve themselves breakfast while you brush your teeth. Overnight oats is like that: it's oatmeal you don't have to cook. We make this one serving at a time so kids can fix it themselves in the evening and grab it from the fridge in the morning. This swirly, cinnamony, milky genius of a breakfast treat is more healthful than store-bought cold cereal and nearly as easy for kids to prepare. We like to use eight-ounce mason jars with screw-top lids so that each jar is a single kid-size serving.

Kid's job! Place ½ cup of oats in each of four 8-ounce mason jars. Add ½ cup of milk to each jar, or just enough to cover the oats, then add ½ teaspoon of honey, a pinch of cinnamon, and ½ teaspoon of vanilla to each jar. Sprinkle raisins into each jar, then give the oats a good stir. Tailor it so it's perfect for each person . . . is there anything special you want to add?

Screw on the lids and let your oats "sleep" in the fridge overnight, or at least six hours.

Breakfast Popsicles

When West and Maison wanted to add scrambled eggs to a popsicle, we bit our tongues and encouraged them to go for it. We realize this is not the behavior of sane people but we've found that saying yes and giving kids license to experiment in the kitchen has been central to reinventing our family's relationship with food. We have a moral responsibility to warn you, if you go this route, there will be some food waste and there will be gastronomic flops. Your kids will likely make pancakes that are leaden, blackish green, and inedible by all accounts. In the process, your kids will also learn about ingredients, textures, and flavors, and there's a good chance they'll become more adventurous when it comes to tasting new foods.

West and Maison thought their breakfast creation was divine. We found it revolting. We can't recommend making these at home—unless you want a breakfast that'll haunt you till the day you die.

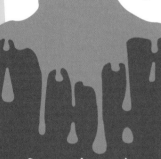

2 cups pineapple chunks

1 kale leaf, stemmed

1 strip bacon, cooked

2 cooked scrambled eggs, cooled

1½ cups orange juice

1 tablespoon maple syrup

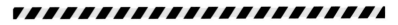

Throw everything into the blender. Blend until smooth. Pour into popsicle molds. Freeze for 4 to 5 hours.

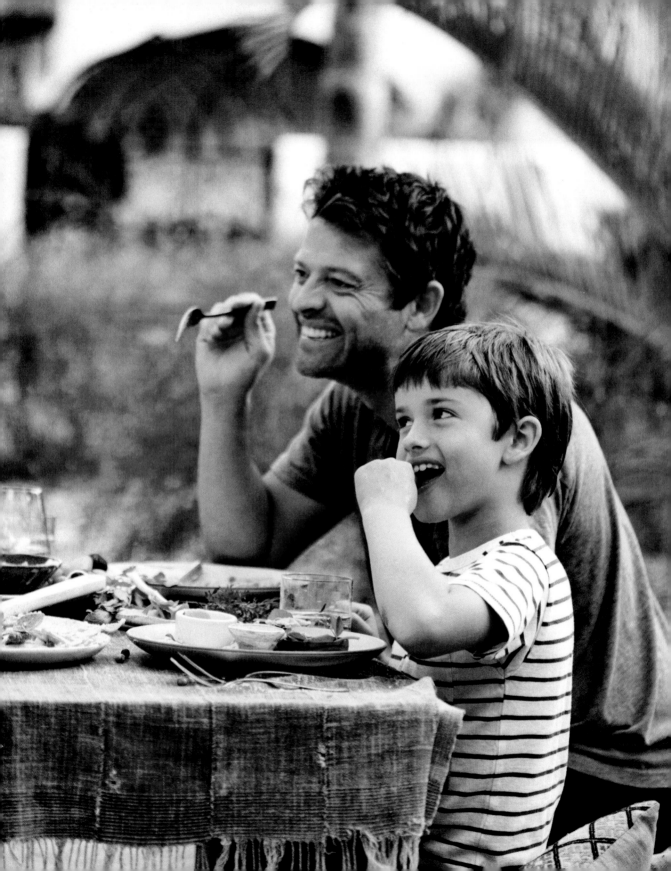

ONE VEGGIE
AT A TIME

Why do many American parents find it so unimaginable that kids would pine for leafy greens or roasted beets? Maybe we've bought into the myth that kids are only capable of enjoying "kids' foods" like burgers and grilled cheese. Maybe some of us are spooked by the memory of mushy canned peas that we were served (and hated) as kids. Who would be excited to eat that?

The truth is, vegetables can be finger-licking good, and children can love them. Our belief is that veggies don't need to be sneaked into muffins or doused in ranch dressing to appeal to kids. Farm-fresh, seasonal produce is becoming more readily available, and there are so many ways to prepare vegetables. Obviously, kids aren't eager to consume bland, overcooked, soggy broccoli. A blanched garden-fresh carrot is a different story.

Consider one of the most controversial members of the Brassicaceae family: cauliflower. Over-boiled into a gooey white pile, it tastes like wet mittens. And yet. The first time Misha roasted cauliflower with a light sheen of olive oil and sea salt, he pulled the florets out of the oven, set them on the counter, then left the kitchen to take a phone call. The kids dragged their stools over and inhaled them all before he got back.

As parents, we can usher our offspring into the wonderful world of vegetables by keeping it simple. A complex vegetable medley can be overwhelming to young children. Giving novice veggie eaters a chance to get to know one veggie at a time is a useful strategy for expanding kids' palates. At first, serve single vegetables with a clear, simple flavor. We keep the seasoning light so the real flavor comes through. Often we dress veggies simply with butter or olive oil, salt, and lemon juice.

That's what this chapter is all about—discovering vegetables, one at a time—and having fun along the way. We hope these recipes inspire your family to experiment with veggies raw, sautéed, steamed, roasted, simmered, and pureed. Here are some of our favorite single-veg recipes to charm the whole family.

THE POWER OF STORY

The stories we tell children about food matter. A study illustrates the power of story when it comes to children's taste. Three groups of kids were all given an unfamiliar vegetable, kohlrabi, for the first time. One group was told a story about a kid who didn't like veggies. The story included the veggie-slamming refrain: "At least the boy didn't have to eat kohlrabi." The second group heard almost the same story, but it featured a positive refrain: "Almost as good as kohlrabi." The last group heard no story. In the second group, two-thirds of the kids who tasted kohlrabi liked it. The only kids who refused to eat it were the ones who heard the negative story. The upshot: share positive messages about foods. Furthermore, it's common for children's books to cast vegetables in an unfavorable light. Chuck books that feature veggie-hating characters and refrains about broccoli tasting yucky. Stories are powerful tools. Can you think of a food you love eating now but it took you time to begin to like it? Tell your kids about it.

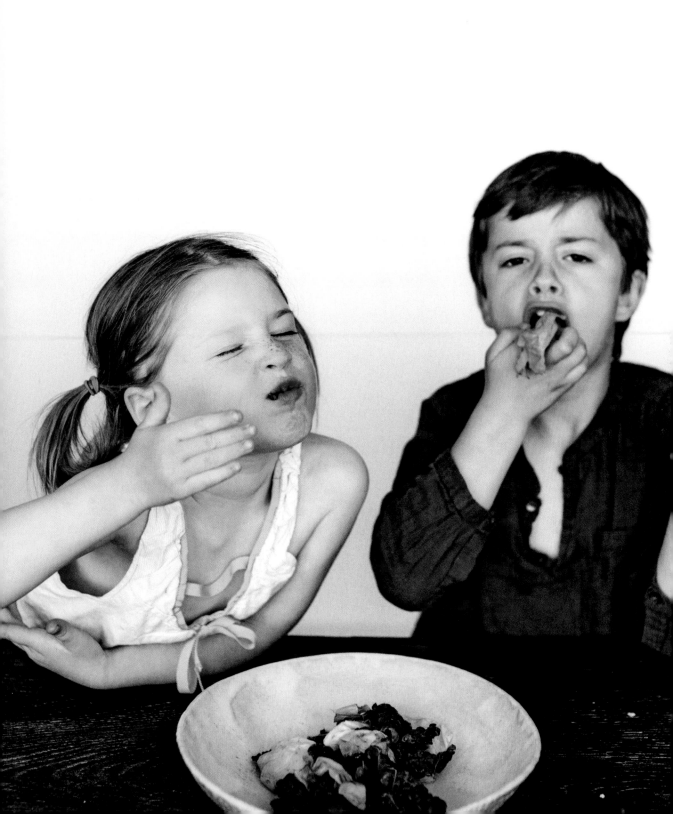

TRIPLE PEA PASTA

SERVES 4

2½ cups shelled fresh peas (from about two pounds pods) or thawed frozen peas

About 6 cups dried pasta (we like to use bow ties for this dish)

3 tablespoons freshly squeezed lemon juice (from about 1½ lemons), divided

¾ cup olive oil, divided

Sea salt to taste

1 cup grated Parmesan cheese, plus more for serving

1 cup fresh pea shoots, roughly chopped (optional)

½ clove garlic

Most children find pasta easy to love. This recipe uses pasta as the gateway for introducing one simple green veggie in three incarnations: peas, pea shoots, and pea sauce. We grow peas in our garden, and our kids spend hours out there, plucking pods off the vine and gobbling the peas. West and Maison find fresh peas irresistible. This recipe is simple and showcases the flavor of peas in a way that rookie pea eaters will appreciate. It's tastiest when fresh peas are in season.

Kid's job! Calling all tiny hands: get to work shelling those peas.

Meanwhile, bring a large pot of salted water to boil. Cook the pasta according to the package directions, then use a slotted spoon or strainer to scoop it out into a big bowl. Keep the pasta water boiling!

While the pasta is still warm, combine it with 2 tablespoons lemon juice, ¼ cup olive oil, and a big sprinkle of salt.

Boil the fresh peas in the pasta water for one minute—when they turn bright green and float, they're done. (Frozen peas won't float—so fish 'em out when they're hot.) Drain, then add 2 cups of peas to the pasta mixture along with the Parmesan and pea shoots.

Combine the remaining peas, 1 tablespoon lemon juice, the remaining ½ cup of olive oil, the garlic, and ¼ cup of water in a blender. Add salt. Blend until ultrasmooth.

Add the pea sauce to the pasta mixture and toss to coat. Serve with extra Parm on the side.

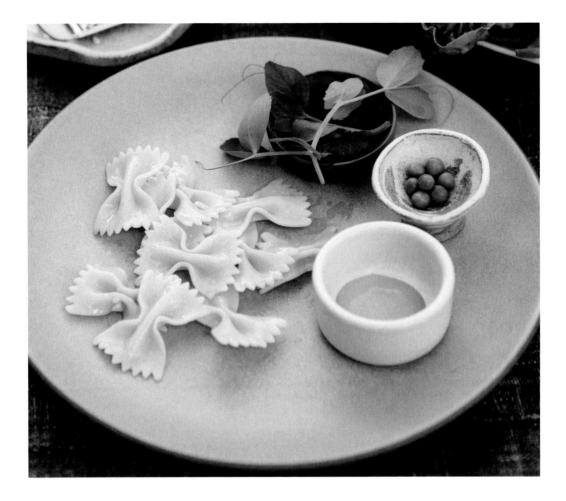

GOTTA KEEP 'EM SEPARATE!

Deconstruct this dish. You can serve it as its component parts: that way, kids can mix them together (or not), which gives hesitant eaters a little more control. For example, instead of adding the peas to the cooked pasta, keep them separate. Serve the peas alongside the pasta in a tiny soy sauce dipping bowl (page 38) with a little butter on top. This way, kids can sample the peas first and then mix them into the pasta if they wish. Pour the green sauce into a separate tiny dipping bowl next to your child's plate—this way she can dip as much as she wants. Pea shoots go in yet another little dipping bowl to taste and sprinkle on as a topper. The final mini bowl is filled with grated Parm to either mix in or sprinkle on top of the pasta.

PURPLE SOUP

SERVES 6

2 tablespoons butter

½ cup roughly chopped yellow onion

2 medium raw beets (about 8 ounces total), roughly chopped (about 1½ cups)

2 medium yellow potatoes (about 12 ounces total), roughly chopped (about 1½ cups)

1 large carrot, roughly chopped (about 1 cup)

Sea salt to taste

4 cups water

1 to 2 tablespoons freshly squeezed lemon juice

Sour cream for garnish

Ad agencies use bright colors to attract kids to junk-food packaging. As parents, we might as well use the vibrant natural colors of fresh vegetables to lure kids, too. This purple soup is the perfect introduction to beets for kids who need a smooth, easy texture. Plus it's fun to decorate with a white sour cream swirl.

Melt the butter in a medium pot over medium heat. Toss in the onion and cook until softened, about 5 to 6 minutes. Add your chopped veggies, salt, and water and bring to a boil over high heat. Cover, reduce heat to low, and simmer 25 to 30 minutes, or until the beets are very soft.

Let the soup cool slightly before pouring it from the pot into a blender. Blend until ultrasmooth and purple.

Return the blended soup to the pot and add the lemon juice. Stir and adjust the seasoning. Serve the soup in mugs or 6-ounce ramekins.

Kid's job! Swirl in sour cream to create a purple fuchsia cyclone.

INVENTORS' CIRCLE

Experiment with Single-Veggie Soups

Karen Le Billon, author and mother of two, spent a year in France trying to pry open her children's palates. She found that pureed single-veggie soups were an effective way to introduce her carb-loving kids to new vegetables. She'd use only one or two primary ingredients in a simple smooth soup, so the flavor of the veggies would come through, and she would serve it with some salted butter and toast. Let your kids pick a veggie that they're game to try in a smooth soup, and invent your recipe together.

TINY TREES IN A GIANT'S BOWL

SERVES 4 TO 6

2 bunches broccoli (about 2 pounds total), trimmed to look like miniature trees

¼ cup (4 tablespoons) unsalted butter

½ teaspoon sea salt

I teaspoon fish sauce

The first time we served broccoli to Maison, we put it in a giant family-size bowl and talked about the tiny trees. This piqued Maison's curiosity. "Do giants eat trees?" She gleefully pretended to be a giant as she devoured a forest of tiny trees. Ever since, we've presented broccoli as tiny trees in a giant's bowl. Broccoli is Maison's comfort food. We recently learned the secret to making broccoli irresistible from a dad friend who owns a local restaurant. Now when we serve it, kids ages three to twelve wolf down the broccoli jungle and beg for more. If your kid is new to broccoli, serve one tiny broccoli tree.

Bring about an inch of water to a boil in a large pot. Add the broccoli, lower the heat to a simmer, cover, and cook for 5 to 6 minutes, or until bright green. The stalks should be soft enough to poke a fork through. Drain well.

In the biggest bowl you have, combine the hot broccoli, salt, fish sauce, and butter, tossing the broccoli and shaking the bowl to melt the butter. Serve.

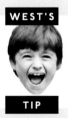

WEST'S

TIP

Eat with Giant Utensils!

The funnest way to eat tiny trees is with giant utensils. How about giant wooden serving spoons? Or extra-large kitchen tongs? Now pretend to be a *giant*.

FAMILY CHALLENGE

Eat a Rainbow

Families thrive when they eat five colors every day. Kids: what's your favorite color? Can you think of a dinner that's made entirely of your favorite color (without any food coloring)? Write down your ideas for each color of the rainbow.

DON'T TOUCH MY BRUSSELS SPROUTS!

SERVES 4 TO 6

3 strips bacon

8 ounces (about 2 cups) brussels sprouts

Sea salt to taste

½ teaspoon maple syrup

In the bad old days, brussels sprouts were served (excessively) boiled, and now they're usually relegated to the kids-find-them-gross category. But our kids have been known to fight over them. Yours probably will, too, if the sprouts are roasted with bacon.

Preheat the oven to 375°F.

Place the bacon on a sheet pan lined with tin foil and bake for 15 to 20 minutes. Transfer the cooked bacon to a paper-towel-lined plate to further crisp and cool. Reserve the rendered bacon fat.

While the bacon is cooking, trim the roots from your pile of brussels sprouts and cut them in half. Arrange the sprouts on the sheet pan and toss to coat them in bacon fat. Sprinkle with salt. Put the pan back in the oven and roast for 12 minutes, or until the sprouts are tender.

Remove the sprouts from the oven. Crumble the bacon over the sprouts, then drizzle with maple syrup. Stir, taste, and add salt to taste. Stir again and serve.

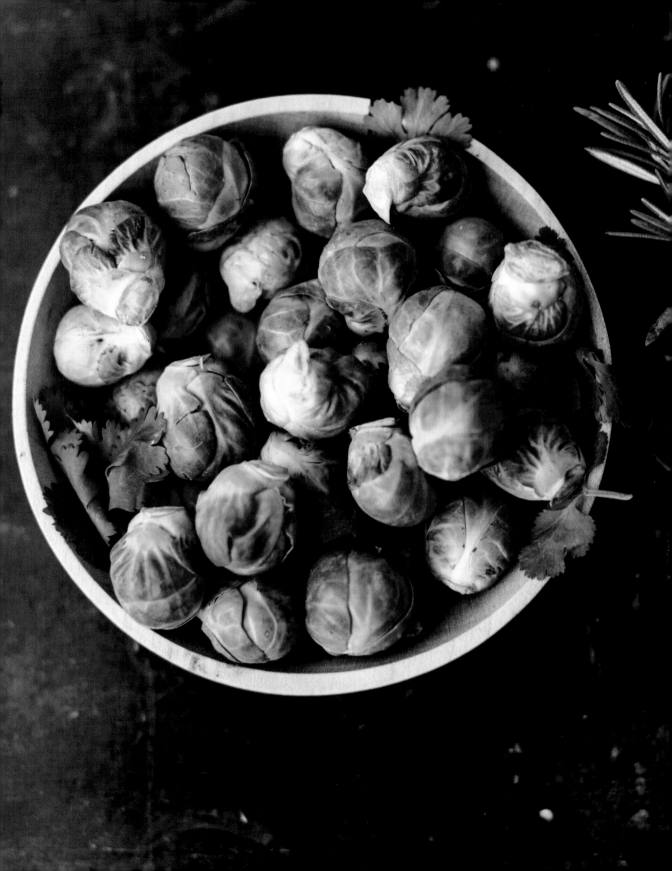

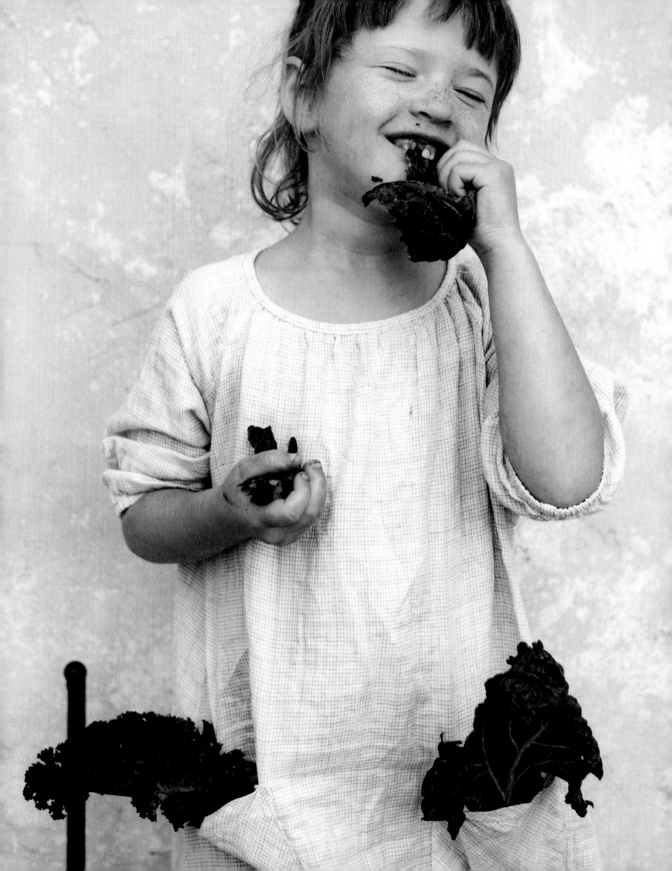

KING OF KALE

SERVES 4 TO 6

2 bunches kale, preferably dino kale, destemmed and thinly sliced

2 to 3 tablespoons olive oil

1 clove garlic

¼ teaspoon sea salt

1 tablespoon balsamic vinegar

¼ teaspoon maple syrup

We have to come clean about our biases. Our family is unflinchingly pro-kale. We've been known to fashion hats from kale leaves and to slither through kale gardens on our bellies. The kale love runs deep. There are many varieties out there, from dark purple to bright green. The mildly flavored curly green variety is the most common. Lacinato kale, or dino kale, is one of our favorites. It's got narrow deep-green leaves with wrinkled bumps. Red Russian is the loud eldest sister of the kale family, with red stems and green leaves; it's sweet with a touch of spice. This is one of our favorite intro-to-kale recipes—an easy kale sauté.

Kid's job! Wash and dry the kale. Hold the stem at the bottom, like a handle, in one hand. Then use your other hand to tear the leaves away from the stem in one swoop. Set aside the stems or use them for a duel. Ask your sous chef parent to thinly slice the kale leaves. Smash the clove of garlic. Let a grown-up mince it!

Add the olive oil to a large skillet over medium heat. Add the garlic and stir constantly. Don't let the garlic brown—it will turn bitter, and that is *not* delicious—so chase it around the pan to keep it moving.

As soon as the garlic sizzles, add the kale, balsamic vinegar, maple syrup, and salt. Stir constantly until the kale is wilted, about 7 minutes.

Serve warm.

CAULIFLOWER MASH

SERVES 4 TO 6

1 small head cauliflower (about 3 heaping cups florets)

1 tablespoon butter, melted

2 tablespoons warm milk

Sea salt to taste

½ cup grated Cheddar or Parmesan cheese

When it comes to sampling a new food, texture is important to kids—they will rule something out before they can even really taste it if it feels the slightest bit weird in their mouths. This creamy cauliflower puree is especially appealing to kids who pine for a smooth, consistent texture.

Trim the leaves and most of the stem from the cauliflower. Pull apart the florets or cut them into pieces of uniform size so they all cook at the same speed.

Bring about an inch of water to a boil in a pot equipped with a steamer basket and a tight-fitting lid. Add the cauliflower to the basket and cover the pot. Lower the heat to a simmer and cook for 5 to 7 minutes, until fork-tender.

Combine the cooked florets, butter, milk, and salt in a blender or food processor. Blend until smooth. If your blender has a wand attachment, use it to help the puree along; otherwise, stop occasionally and scrape down the sides of the container with a spatula. When your puree is smooth, taste and adjust seasoning. Spoon into bowls, top with grated cheese, and serve warm.

EXPERTS SAY

INVITE THE **WHOLE FAMILY** TO THE **VEGGIE PARTY**

- Welcome kids into the kitchen. Let them grate carrots or destem kale. Being part of the food-prep process elicits curiosity, pride, and ownership—all of which makes kids more willing to take a bite.

- Serve *tiny*, *tiny*, *tiny* portions of new foods (we're talking four peas, parents) so kids don't get overwhelmed. They can always ask for more.

- Try out a new vegetable next to foods kids are already familiar with. Dinner = one unfamiliar plant-based item + two to three familiar foods. If your kids aren't up for tasting the new item on the plate, no biggie. Exposing them to the sight, smell, and texture of the veggie will increase their familiarity with it and ultimately can lead to their tasting it (and loving it) down the road.

- Be patient and persistent—keep exposing your kids to diverse veggies, even if they don't immediately go for them and regardless of what they say or whether they eat them. It can take fifteen tries (or more!) before a kid accepts a new food, and most parents in the US give up after two attempts.

- Now, here's the really tricky part . . . don't pressure, and for the love of all that is crispy and green, don't even comment on whether your kid decided to let said veggie touch his lips. Don't coerce, cajole, threaten, bribe, or sweet-talk your kid into tasting anything he's not ready to try. Pretty please don't extol its health virtues. All these forms of pressure tend to backfire by inadvertently intensifying veggie resistance.

- Try various temperatures and prep methods for veggies. If your kid won't touch a fresh green bean, it doesn't mean everything green is off-limits. Asparagus, for example, smells one way when it's raw and another way when it's cooked. If your kid is sensitive to smell, try serving cauliflower, broccoli, and cabbage raw for a mellower aroma.

- Once your kid has decided she likes a particular veggie, explore other ways to prepare it. If raw carrots are her thing, try cutting them into matchsticks one day and curls the next. Just changing the cut can be a useful step toward opening children up to new foods.

- Make sure kids come to the table hungry. A satiated kid isn't going to be eager to try anything new. Cut off snacking two hours before mealtime.

- Serve vegetables as the first course. Preschoolers served veggies first ate 47 percent more of them, according to the *American Journal of Clinical Nutrition*.

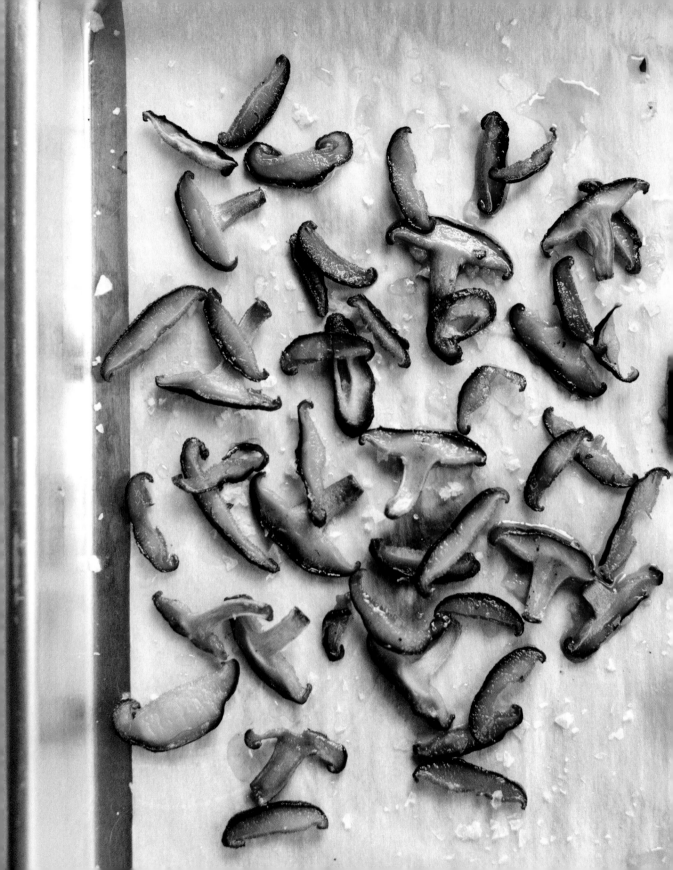

SHIITAKE CRISPIES

SERVES 4 TO 6

4 ounces shiitake
mushrooms
(about 25 small)

¼ cup olive oil

Generous pinch of
sea salt to taste

A rookie mistake a lot of parents make is serving up mushrooms that are slimy. Yes, we call it sautéed, and we know that oil, garlic, and onions add to a mushroom's deliciousness, but kids just see slickness, and for them that can be the difference between loving mushrooms and hating them. Again, with kids, it's often all about texture. When it comes to mushrooms, think crispy and salty. Even fledgling mushroom eaters might be tempted to taste these crispy bites.

Preheat the oven to 400°F.

Kid's job! A little dirt never hurt. To clean mushrooms, dampen a paper towel and wipe away any excess dirt.

Slice the mushroom caps thinly—really, *really* thinly. Half an inch. (Caps only; discard the stems.) In a large bowl, toss the sliced mushrooms, oil, and salt. Coat all the slices well.

Spread the mushrooms out in a single layer on a parchment-lined sheet pan. Give your mushrooms plenty of room—you want them to crisp; if they don't have enough space between them, they'll steam.

Bake for 20 minutes without stirring. Let cool slightly, then nibble straight from the pan.

SNOW-CAPPED ARTICHOKES

SERVES 4

4 medium artichokes

I lemon, halved

I cup unseasoned
bread crumbs

¼ cup olive oil

Pinch of sea salt

¼ cup grated Cheddar
cheese

¼ cup grated Monterey
Jack cheese

¼ cup grated Parmesan
cheese

2 to 4 ounces Brie
cheese, sliced, rind
removed

Melted butter
for dipping

Artichokes are easy for kids to love. Maybe it's the fun of pulling off the leaves? Or the way you have to wrestle the goodness out of them? Or the industriousness required to extract the heart? To make them even more tantalizing, we top the 'chokes with various cheeses to create a melted-cheese taste test.

Lop off the pointy top of each artichoke to make a flat top.

Fill an oven-safe pot (one that's small enough to keep the artichokes upright) with half an inch of water. Place the artichokes in the pot stem side down and squeeze the lemon halves over them. Add the squeezed halves to the pot. Cover with a lid and cook over medium-high heat for 35 minutes, checking occasionally to make sure the water doesn't steam off—add more water if needed.

After 35 minutes, pull off a leaf and taste it. You want the artichokes to be very tender. Keep steaming in five-minute increments as needed. Depending on the size of your artichokes, you might need to steam for up to 45 minutes.

Once the artichokes are tender, turn on your broiler.

Kid's job! Combine the bread crumbs, olive oil, and salt in a small bowl. Sprinkle a couple of spoonfuls of the bread-crumb mixture onto each artichoke. Work the bread crumbs in between the leaf layers with your fingers. It's okay to get a little messy.

Top one of the artichokes with the Cheddar, another with the Monterey Jack, another with the Parmesan, and another with the Brie. Place the pot under the broiler for 2 to 3 minutes, or until the cheese is melted and bubbling.

Serve with a dish of melted butter on the side for leaf dipping. Which melted cheese tastes best on the artichoke? Take a poll at the table.

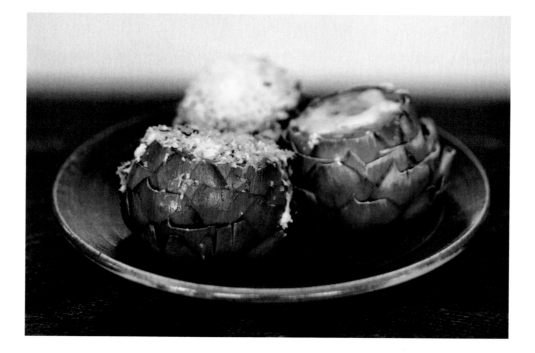

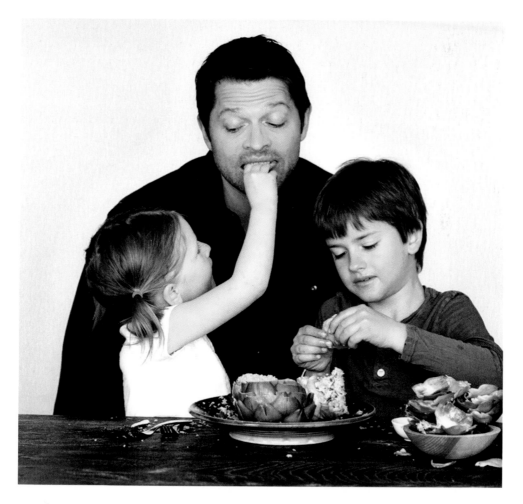

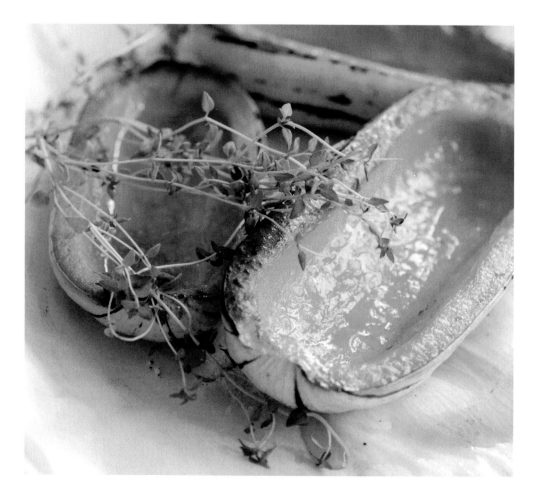

TURN THE SEEDS
INTO A CRUNCHY SNACK

Stick your fingers in the goop. Scoop the goop! Pull out all the strings and seeds with your hands. Toss all the goop and seeds into a bowl of water. Using your fingers, separate the seeds from the strings, letting the stringy stuff float and the seeds sink. Use your eagle eyes to find any little strings and pull them off every seed. Dump them onto a clean kitchen towel to dry off, then transfer them to a sheet pan.

Preheat your oven to 325°F. Drizzle olive oil and salt over the seeds, and spread them into a single layer. Bake for 20 to 30 minutes, stirring every 10 minutes. When the seeds are dry and crisp, remove them from the oven. Add more salt and serve.

DELICATA BOATS

SERVES 4

1 delicata squash, about 1½ pounds

2 tablespoons olive oil

2 tablespoons butter, divided

2 tablespoons maple syrup, divided

Sea salt to taste

We like to roast these striped squash to bring out their rich flavor and natural sweetness, then supplement with a little maple syrup. Once your kids decide they love squash, you can fill the hollows with various ingredients. To get them started, try this simple recipe.

Preheat the oven to 400°F.

Rinse and dry the squash. Halve the squash lengthwise and scoop out the seeds and goop. Rub each half all over with olive oil, then lay the halves cut side down on a sheet pan lined with parchment paper. Bake for 40 minutes.

Once the squash halves are tender, remove them from the oven and flip them over. Fill each hollow with 1 tablespoon butter and 1 tablespoon maple syrup, then sprinkle with salt. Cut each half in half. Serve with a spoon (and probably a bib).

KEEP CALM AND KEEP SERVING VEGGIES

Whatever you do, when serving kids veggies, do not panic. Every parent knows that children can smell fear. Once they get a whiff of your fear, they'll gain the upper hand. You're cooking vegetables with (and for) your child—you are not going into battle. Food can be an arena of joy, discovery, and connection. As parents, we can get so stressed about what our kids are or aren't eating. Instead of getting caught up in the tense will-my-child-eat-this drama, focus on the delicious meal you're preparing with your family. Taste the vegetable. Does it need more butter? More salt? A squeeze of lemon juice? Remember: your job is to provide food. If your kid isn't up for tasting a veggie you've prepared, don't fret. Whether or not your kid eats the food is up to them. Bravo to you for putting a new veggie on the table. Keep enjoying your veggies, and keep serving them. One day, your kid might start enjoying them right alongside you.

ROASTED ROOTS

Roasting at high heat totally changes a vegetable's flavor, texture, and smell. Our kids love to scrub root veggies and snip their favorite herbs to throw them into the root roast. We like to use fresh rosemary, lavender, and tarragon. When roasted veggies come out of the oven, our kids often nab them off the pan before we can get them onto plates. Let kids choose which roots to taste. Roasted roots might win your reluctant eaters over. Here are a few ideas to get you started . . .

HEARTBEETS

SERVES 4

2 to 3 medium raw red beets, scrubbed, peeled, and sliced ½ inch thick

2 to 3 medium purple potatoes, scrubbed, peeled, and sliced ½ inch thick

2 to 3 leaves fresh sage, chopped

1 tablespoon olive oil

Sea salt to taste

Kid's job! Scrub and peel the roots. Let a grown-up slice the beets and potatoes. Once sliced, use cookie cutters to cut them into hearts, stars, and whatever you please.

Preheat the oven to 375°F.

Combine the beets, potatoes, and sage in a large bowl. Drizzle with olive oil and season with plenty of salt. Toss to coat, then spread in a single layer on a sheet pan. Roast for 35 to 45 minutes, tossing the veggies halfway through.

BUNNY SPICE

SERVES 4

3 cups ½-inch-thick carrot slices

3 cups ½-inch-thick parsnip slices

1 tablespoon olive oil

Sea salt to taste

1 teaspoon cinnamon

Preheat the oven to 375°F.

Combine carrots, parsnips, dill, and cinnamon in a large bowl. Drizzle with olive oil and season with plenty of salt. Toss to coat, then spread in a single layer on a sheet pan. Roast for 35 to 45 minutes, rotating the pan halfway through.

MISHA GETS ROMANTIC WITH ROOTS

When I asked Vicki to marry me, years ago, I brought her to a windy beach in Maine. I served her a picnic with roasted pumpkin and parsnip. It was early October and the smell of roasted roots still reminds me of that sweet time. I'll spoil the ending—she said yes. I credit the parsnips.

CELEBRATE THE VEGGIE, DON'T SNEAK IT

Avocado has always been entirely off-limits for our son. It was his first food as a baby, and he puked after eating it. To this day, he doesn't like it. (Our daughter, on the other hand, could eat an avocado every day.) At some point, West might taste an avocado and love it—who knows? For now, we know he doesn't eat it, and we don't push it— usually.

But one day a friend made a divine smoothie that contained some avocado. It had been a long, long time since West had willingly tried avocado, so we figured we'd let him taste the smoothie without revealing the secret ingredient. He instantly identified the offending flavor. When we confessed, he was pissed. To punish us, he insisted on getting an exhaustive ingredients list for every food on his plate for weeks after. We swore never again to sneak him avocado. He's certain that we're still secretly slipping trace amounts of avocado into his dinner.

"If you're dishonest with your children about their food, they become suspicious, cautious, and reluctant to try new food," says kids'-food guru Ellyn Satter. Turns out, most kid-food pros don't recommend sneaking veggies (or other healthful ingredients) into kids' meals. This can feel like a breach of trust to kids. Ideally, we want food to be an area of trust, fun, and joy in our family. Plus, stuffing pureed spinach into a Pop-Tart probably won't foster a welcoming attitude toward new foods or a love of veggies. So celebrate the veggie—play with it, wear it as a hat, sing to it. Please don't sneak it into the meal or disguise it as something it isn't.

LOVELY LEEKS AND POTATOES

SERVES 4

3 large leeks (white part only)

3 cups halved new potatoes

2 tablespoons roughly chopped fresh rosemary

1 clove garlic, minced

1 tablespoon olive oil

Sea salt to taste

Preheat the oven to 375°F.

Kid's job! Once the leeks are trimmed of the green parts and cut in half, dunk them in a bowl of cold water. Jiggle them until all the dirt shakes out. Clean leeks are tastier.

Slice each half into ½-inch half-moons. You should have around 3 cups.

Combine the leeks, potatoes, rosemary, and garlic in a large bowl. Drizzle with olive oil and season with plenty of salt. Toss to coat, then spread in a single layer on a sheet pan. Roast for 35 to 45 minutes, tossing the veggies halfway through.

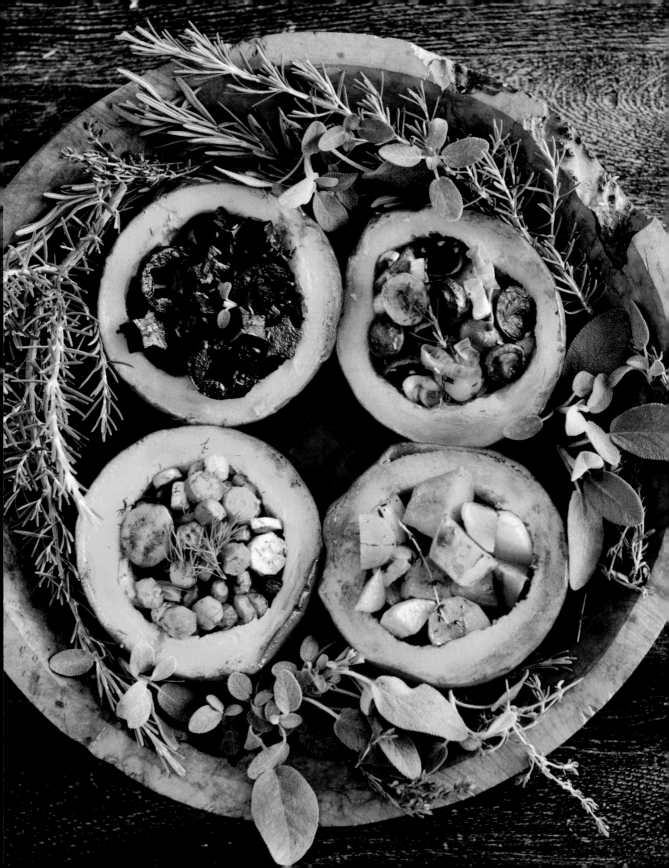

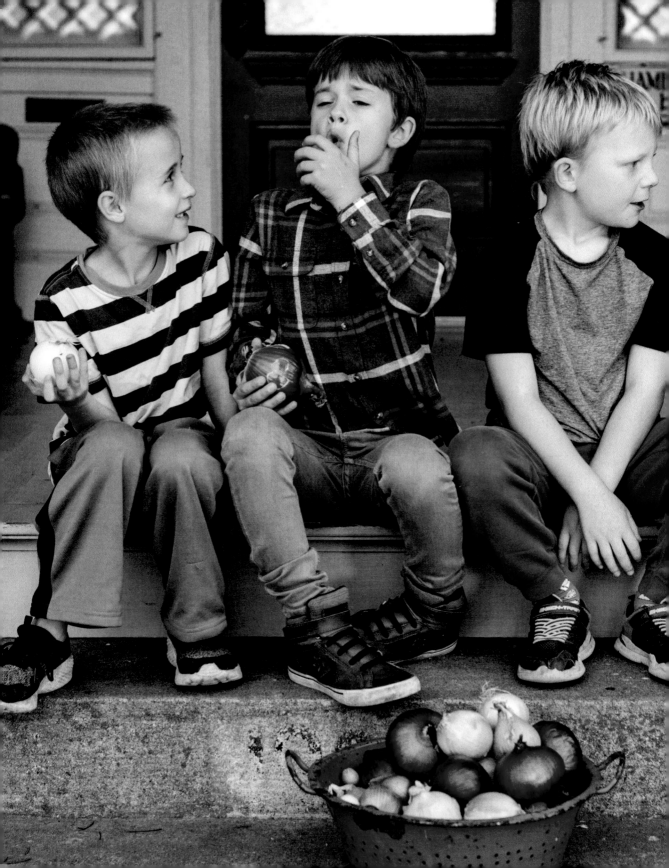

ADVENTURES IN ONIONS

Many American parents have concluded that kids don't like onions, so we're dedicating an entire mini chapter to them. To be honest, our kids did not welcome onions into their lives with open mouths. They eyed onions of all types dubiously—even onion rings were suspect. Ever vigilant in his guard against intrusive ingredients, West would meticulously inspect each meal with a fervor normally reserved for crime scene investigations and ferret out any nearly invisible onion sliver that may have touched his grain of rice. We did what any parent would do in that situation—we leaped to the rescue by removing the offending onion in hopes that it would soon be forgotten and the meal would continue unaffected.

In the spring of 2018, something shifted. Finally. The chives we planted in our garden were the only plants to survive the Pacific Northwest winter. We told West and Maison that the purple puffy flowers on top are edible—they were skeptical. They got to work with their scissors, snipping the chives. Maison noted that the snipped chives looked like green elf brace-lets. We spread the purple blossoms and green chives that they'd harvested out on the table alongside little dishes of cream cheese, crackers, sour cream, and Parmesan slivers. Maison posed a provocative question: How do elf bracelets taste on cream cheese? Hmm . . . they were curious. West nibbled a blossom. This was a milestone: West, at age eight, intentionally consumed part of an onion.

Now West and Maison nosh on raw chives from the garden, and they're spreading the word in their kid circles that onions can be tasty. When West's friend Atticus balked at onions, West said, "Why? Onions are delicious." Bowing to peer pressure, Atticus gave it a taste and reported, "Hmm. Pretty good." Maison even added chives to waffle batter once—which we can't, in good faith, endorse—but we're excited that she and West have started down the path of onion appreciation.

Our favorite onion-tasting recipes are laid out below in order of difficulty level, beginning with what we found to be the friendliest gateway onion—chives.

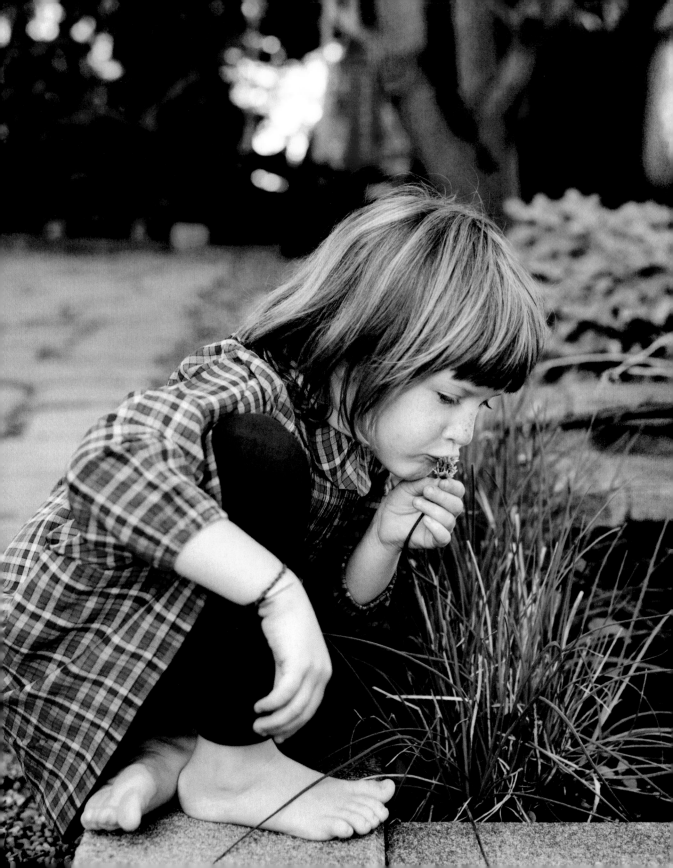

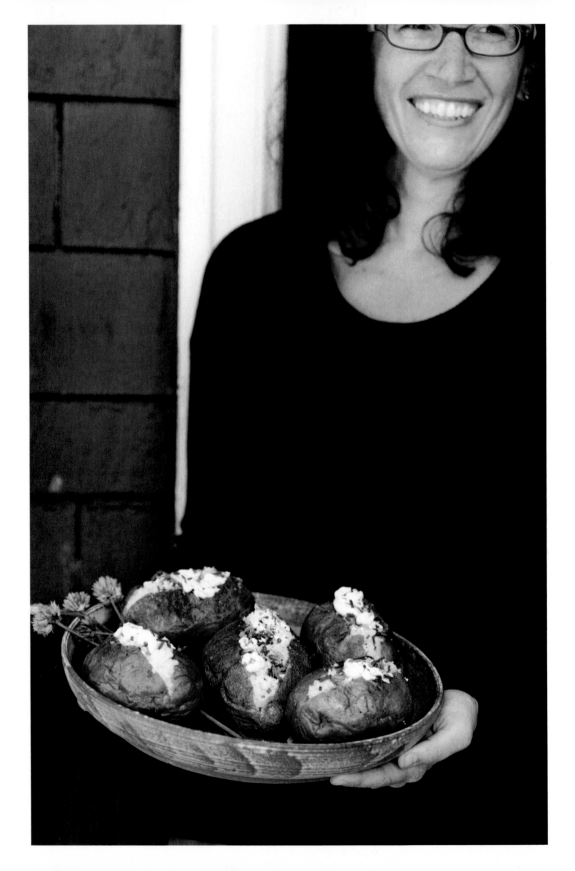

PARTY POTATOES

SERVES 4

4 unpeeled medium russet potatoes (about 20 ounces total), scrubbed

2 tablespoons olive oil

Sea salt to taste

TOPPINGS

¼ cup (4 tablespoons) butter, divided

¼ cup sour cream

2 tablespoons snipped or minced fresh chives

8 to 10 fresh chive blossoms (optional)

¼ cup popped popcorn (optional)

When we were kids (*waaaaay* back in the long-ago '80s), baked potatoes were a staple of the dinner table. Then the fear-of-carbs trend hit and drove these scrumptious tubers into obscurity. The truth: potatoes are delicious and healthful (potassium, fiber, protein!). They also make a perfect canvas for onions, letting kids tiptoe into that world of flavor. Simply top a baked potato with sour cream, butter, and fresh chives. Oniony bliss.

Preheat the oven to 425°F.

Kid's job! Give those potatoes a bath: scrub your potatoes under running water. Scrub, scrub, scrub. This is more fun with a little veggie brush. If your potato has any sprouting eyes, dig those out with the poky end of a swivel peeler. Pat your potatoes dry with a paper towel.

Using a fork, stab some holes in those potatoes. Rub olive oil all over them with your hands. Things might get slippery, so hold on. Don't let them escape. Sprinkle some salt on top.

Place greased, salted, hole-poked potatoes directly on the oven rack. Bake for 50-ish minutes, flipping them every 20 minutes or so. Stick a fork in them. If the insides are soft and pillowy, they're done.

Halve the potatoes lengthwise and top each with 1 tablespoon butter—use a fork to mash the butter into the potato and help it melt—then sprinkle with more salt. Set the sour cream, chives, and chive blossoms (and even popcorn) out in tiny bowls and let kids top their potatoes as their hearts desire.

GARLIC:
THE ONION'S COUSIN

Depending on how you prepare it, garlic can taste very different. Raw, it's pungent and spicy; slow-roasted, it loses some of its kick and sweetens, like caramelized onions. For kids new to garlic, we like to prep the cloves by smashing them first, which mellows the flavor.

Giving kids a chance to smell, feel, and work with garlic will familiarize them with it. Invite them to experiment with various garlic prep methods.

Kid's job! Give a garlic bulb a good smash with a mallet. Crush as many individual cloves as you plan to use by slapping a small pan on top of each one and pressing down *hard*. Then remove the skin and chop them into tiny pieces using a kid-safe knife.

Alternatively, try West's favorite garlic peeling method: whack a head of garlic with a mallet to break apart the cloves. Put the cloves in a metal bowl. Place another metal bowl over the top of the bowl filled with garlic. Grab hold of the edges of the two bowls and shake them like maracas. Take a look. Garlic is magically peeled!

CHEESY BROWN RICE
WITH LEEKS AND BOK CHOY

SERVES 4

3 baby bok choy
(12 ounces total)

1 tablespoon olive oil

1 leek (white part only),
thinly sliced

1 clove garlic, minced

Sea salt to taste

2½ cups cooked
short-grained brown
or arborio rice

1 tablespoon butter

½ cup grated
Parmesan cheese

As members of the garlic and onion family, leeks have a mild, oniony flavor, which makes for a solid second step up the onion ladder—not too pungent, not too scary. This recipe has a mellow flavor and is so creamy and risottolike you'd swear it took hours to make (it's actually really fast). We've also thrown in bok choy, a mild veggie with a slightly crunchy texture.

Bring a large pot of salted water to a boil. Add the bok choy and cook until it's bright green, about 1 minute. Use a slotted spoon or tongs to transfer it into a colander to drain, reserving the cooking water. When the greens are cool enough to handle, use your hands to squeeze any excess water out of them. Roughly chop the bok choy and set aside.

Heat the olive oil in a large pan over medium heat until hot but not smoking. Add the leek and garlic to the pan and sprinkle with salt. Stir constantly until the garlic and leek are softened and fragrant, about 2 minutes. Don't let the garlic burn—adjust the heat as needed.

Turn the heat up to medium-high. Add the bok choy, rice, butter, and 1½ cups of the reserved cooking water to the garlic-leek mixture. Cook, stirring constantly, for a few minutes, until the rice gets nice and creamy. Stir in the grated cheese and another dash of salt and serve.

KIDS ▶ **DO LEEKS MAKE YOU SQUEAK?**

A Roman emperor named Nero ate leeks every day because he believed they improved his singing voice. Test this theory. Sing your favorite tune at the dinner table. Eat some leeky rice. Sing again. Well? Which version sounds better?

FRENCH ONION SOUP
À LA WALLA WALLA

SERVES 4

1½ sticks butter
(12 tablespoons)

4 large Walla Walla or
other sweet onions,
thinly sliced (about
8 cups)

Sea salt to taste

2 tablespoons balsamic
vinegar

2 tablespoons soy sauce

2 quarts beef stock

CROUTONS

4 toasted baguette slices

4 1-ounce slices cheese,
such as Gruyère, Jack,
Cheddar, or Swiss

Heralded for its sweetness, the Walla Walla onion became Washington State's official vegetable in 2007. Walla Walla devotees claim you can bite into this sweet onion raw, like an apple. While our family isn't quite there yet, we do love these onions in our special soup.

Melt the butter in a large pot over medium-high heat. Add the onions and salt and sauté for 20 minutes, stirring only a few times. No need to stir continuously; let the onions hang out and do their thing. Reduce the heat to medium or even medium-low if you see lots of brown color coming on—you want the onions to be translucent, soft, sweet, and a deep golden brown.

Once the onions have started to caramelize and soften up nicely, add the balsamic vinegar, soy sauce, and stock to the pot. Taste and adjust the seasoning, then bring the soup to a simmer.

Meanwhile, top each slice of bread with a slice of cheese and warm them in a toaster oven until the cheese is melted and just a tad brown.

Ladle the hot soup into bowls, float a cheesy crouton cap on each one, and serve.

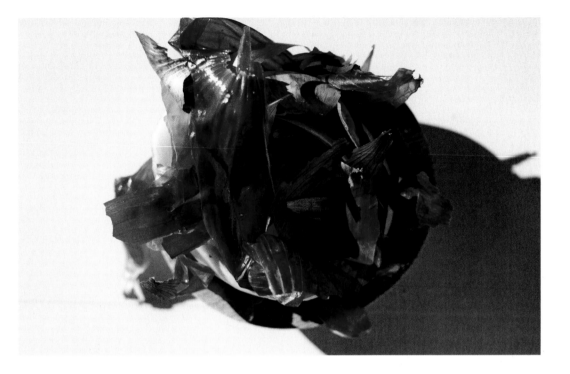

EXPERIMENT: CRY-PROOF ONION CHOPPING

Have you ever noticed that grown-ups sob like babies when they make onion soup? That's because slicing into an onion emits a sulfoxide gas that irritates eyes. Sure, it might be entertaining to watch grown-ups get misty-eyed while they chop onions, but if you're in the mood to be a kitchen hero, use a kid-safe knife and test out the strategies below for ending the sobfest.

Ask a grown-up to cut an onion in half for you—that way it'll stay put, flat side down, while you do your slicing experiment.

Strategy 1. Wear swim goggles or sunglasses while slicing. Does it work? Did you tear up? (There are even onion-cutting goggles on the market, but seriously, who has those?)

Strategy 2. Soak the onion in a cold bath for a few minutes before slicing. Dry it off. Start slicing. Did you cry less?

Strategy 3. Bite on a slice of bread while slicing. Does it work?

If none of these work, invent your own strategy.

FAMILY INTERVIEWS

NEW FOODS CAN BE SCARY
(AND EXCITING)

Join the adventurous eaters club! It takes a lot of guts to try a new food.
Has anyone in your family tasted a new food lately?
Kudos to you for trying something new!

KIDS | Interview Your Parents

What did you like eating as a kid that you don't like eating now?

What's a food you used to dislike that you now enjoy?

How old were you when you first tried that food?

How old were you when you started liking it?

What's your favorite food memory?

What is your funniest food memory?

What's the most surprising thing you've ever eaten?

PARENTS | Interview Your Kids

What's a food you used to not like eating that you like now?

What's the most unusual thing you've ever eaten? What made it unusual?

What's something you were afraid to taste, but then you ate it and liked it?

What's the yummiest thing you've ever eaten?

Keep a record of your family's adventurous eating!

ONION PIE

½ stick (4 tablespoons) butter

3 sweet yellow or white onions, thinly sliced

Sea salt to taste

2 tablespoons all-purpose flour

3 eggs

½ cup sour cream

½ cup grated Gruyère cheese

¼ teaspoon paprika

1 premade 9-inch piecrust

This is one "onionful" dish. Once your kids have started on their onion-appreciation journey, they might be game to try this one. Part quiche, part pie, this dish features onions that have been caramelized into a sweetness that's appealing to both kids and adults. (Our recipe uses a store-bought crust because we usually don't have the bandwidth to make crust from scratch. When Misha was a kid, his mom made this whenever onions were on sale. It's been his comfort food ever since. "The first few times I made it for Vicki, she wrinkled her nose, but I think it's her comfort food now, too (or she just feels sorry for me)," says Misha.

Preheat the oven to 375°F.

Melt the butter in a large skillet over medium heat. Add the onions along with a generous pinch of salt. Cover and cook for 15 minutes, stirring occasionally. Then uncover and cook, still stirring occasionally, until the onions are fully caramelized and a deep golden brown, another 15 minutes. Sprinkle the flour over the onions and stir. Sauté another few minutes, until you see the butter thickening on the onions and beginning to coat them. Remove from the heat and let the onions cool slightly.

Meanwhile, crack the eggs into a bowl and break up the yolks with a whisk. Add the sour cream, cheese, paprika, and a few pinches of salt and whisk until well mixed.

Fold in the onions and pour everything into the crust. Bake for 25 minutes, or until the middle has some jiggle but the rest of the filling has set.

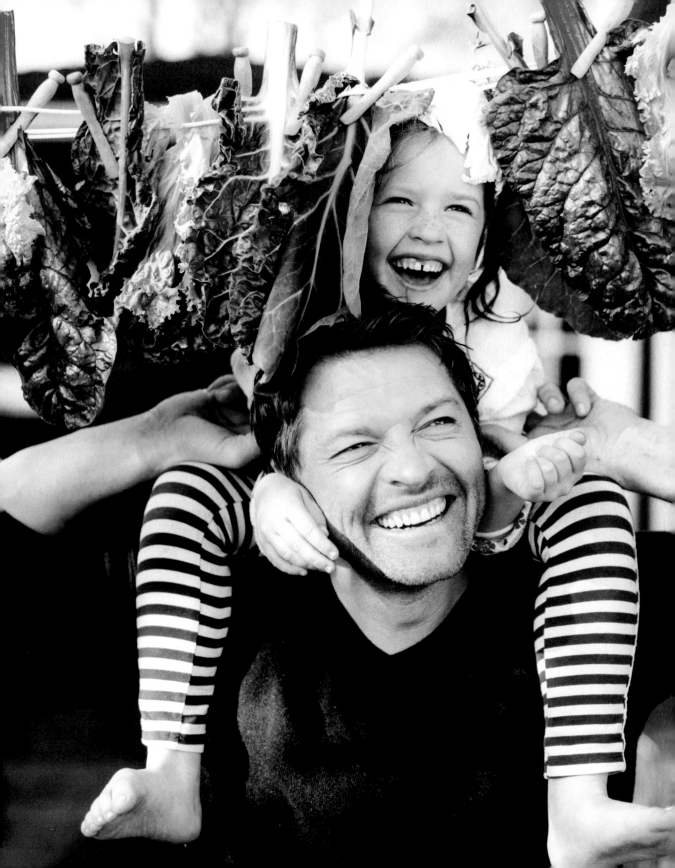

GET YOUR GREEN ON

We all know that salad is good for you, but "Eat it—it's healthy" is a line that doesn't work on kids. In fact, research shows that labeling food "healthy" often makes it *less* enticing to kids. So let's drop the high-and-mighty health spiel and start speaking a language kids can relate to: can salad be irresistibly delicious?

We say *yes*.

Whenever we meet a child who says she doesn't like salad, we're curious. After all, there are millions of ways to make a salad. If a kid's salad experience has been limited to refrigerator-case iceberg lettuce topped with mealy tomatoes and sad, syrupy dressing, it can't come as a surprise that she's not swooning over salad. Has she ever tasted a fresh pea shoot? Or the velvety leaves of butter lettuce? Kids are more likely to fall in love with salad when it's colorful, beautiful, and made with farm-fresh produce.

This might seem like a no-brainer, but often parents dumb down salad for kids—assuming that only a baby carrot smothered in ranch dressing will be acceptable for young palates. Salads are one of the easiest foods for kids to prepare because there's no hot stove involved and the recipe can be as simple or as complex as they want it to be. When kids participate in creating the salad, they have a chance to nibble on ingredients and experience each element on its own. This teaches kids that mixing ingredients together doesn't create a totally unknown new food.

When West has had a hard day, he asks for salad: it's his comfort food. He's been known to polish off an entire serving bowl of salad meant for a family of four. This isn't something we've beaten into him.

We want your kids to love salad as much as ours do, so we put the easy-to-eat salads at the beginning and pushed the challenging ones to the end of the chapter (by which point, we hope, your kids will be salad fanatics).

Before you start serving leafy greens to your kids, have some fun. May we suggest making your own matching family collard-greens slippers?

West's words of encouragement to newbie salad tasters: "If you don't like salad, try it again and again and again and again and you'll probably like it someday, but maybe not."

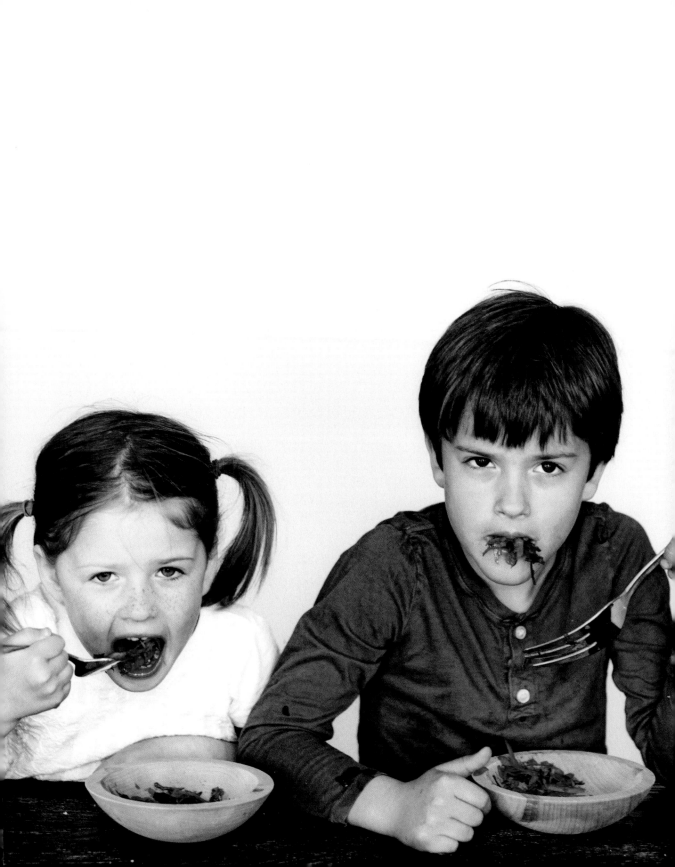

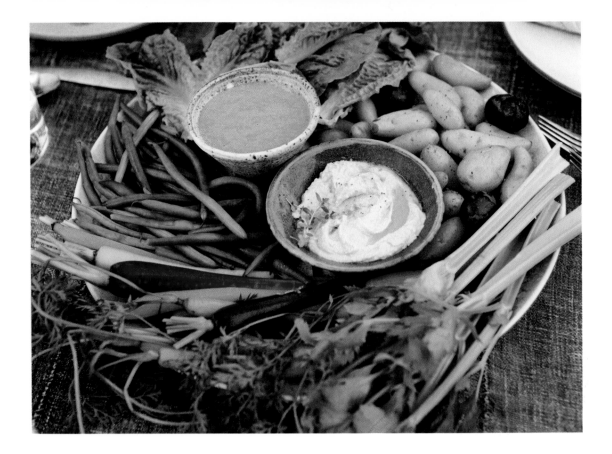

TURN YOUR KID INTO A SALAD LOVER

DIY Salad

If your kids are new to salad, kids'-food experts suggest deconstructing it into its components so they have the chance to taste each ingredient individually first. In other words, if your salad contains shredded beets, lettuce, and dressing, make a tiny pile of beets (like, two shreds), a tiny pile of lettuce (two leaves), and a tiny pile of the mixed salad, plus a tiny dipping bowl of dressing. This approach can work with most of the recipes in this chapter.

If your kid is feeling daring, she might be up for tasting a complicated new dish if she knows she can deconstruct it. Maison has gotten more adventurous when it comes to tasting complex, unfamiliar meals. Her strategy: "I taste the whole thing in one bite, then I think about what I want to pick out to make it a little bit better."

FORK-FREE SALAD

SERVES 4

Choose 2 or 3

Handful of green beans, trimmed

8 ounces asparagus, woody ends trimmed

8 ounces broccoli, separated into florets

Handful of new potatoes

1 head crisp romaine, trimmed, leaves separated

1 bunch rainbow carrots with stems

1 bunch celery with leaves, trimmed, stalks separated

We consider this Salad 101—it's a welcoming starter salad that's perfect for rookie salad eaters because it gives them a sense of control. Kids can pick and choose the veggies they want to try. Another perk for the salad-wary: kids can easily identify all the veggies, since they haven't been chopped into tiny pieces and hidden as they often are in traditional salads.

Crisp, fresh leaves. Entire carrots with stems for handles. It's quite unfussy to prepare: simply wash, trim, and throw the ingredients on a platter. Let your kids choose as many or as few of the veggies as they'd like from the ingredients suggested here. Serve with small bowls of dressing (pages 137–140) for dipping. We like to go *big* on this one, making a giant platter the whole family can share. Kids can often find at least one element in this salad that intrigues them—perhaps enough to taste it or at least to try it on as a mustache. The real bonus: eating a salad with your hands is fun, even for adults.

First, tenderize your veggies. Bring a large pot of water to a rolling boil. As it heats, make an ice bath: fill a large mixing bowl with ice water and set it aside. Immerse the green beans in the boiling water for 10 seconds—you just want them a little tender and bright green.

Using tongs or a large slotted spoon, transfer the beans to the ice bath, which will stop the cooking. When the beans are cool, use tongs to transfer them to a paper-towel-lined plate. Repeat with the asparagus, cooking for 30 to 60 seconds; then repeat with the broccoli, cooking for 45 seconds. The potatoes will take the longest—boil for 12 to 15 minutes, until just fork-tender.

Then assemble your salad. Choose the crispest and longest pieces of romaine for this dish. Arrange the lettuce, carrots, and celery on a platter around your small bowls of dressing. We like to serve this with strawberry dressing, hummus, or a simple vinaigrette. Pile the green beans, asparagus, broccoli, and potatoes around and in between the raw veggies. Enjoy a salad-dipping party.

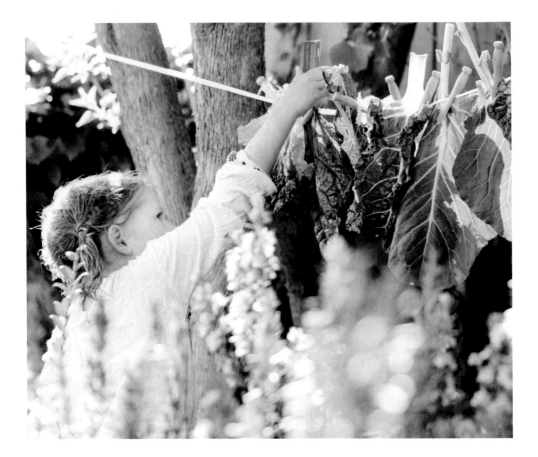

WASH AND DRY YOUR GREENS

To wash your greens or veggies, fill a large bowl or bucket with cold water. Dunk the leafy greens in the water. Give those greens a gentle swirl with your hands to help shake loose any grit and dirt. Let the dirt settle at the bottom of the bowl, then lift out your greens. For extra muddy lettuce, repeat this cold-water dunk two more times with fresh water for squeaky-clean greens. Be gentle so you don't bruise the leaves.

Dry greens are key to a yummy salad because the dressing can really cling to them—so get those greens really dry. Pat them with a clean dish towel or give 'em a whirl in a salad spinner. West loves pumping the salad spinner. Spin those greens till they are superdry. Or try our old-fashioned drying method . . . hang the greens outside on a clothesline to dry in the sun for 10 minutes.

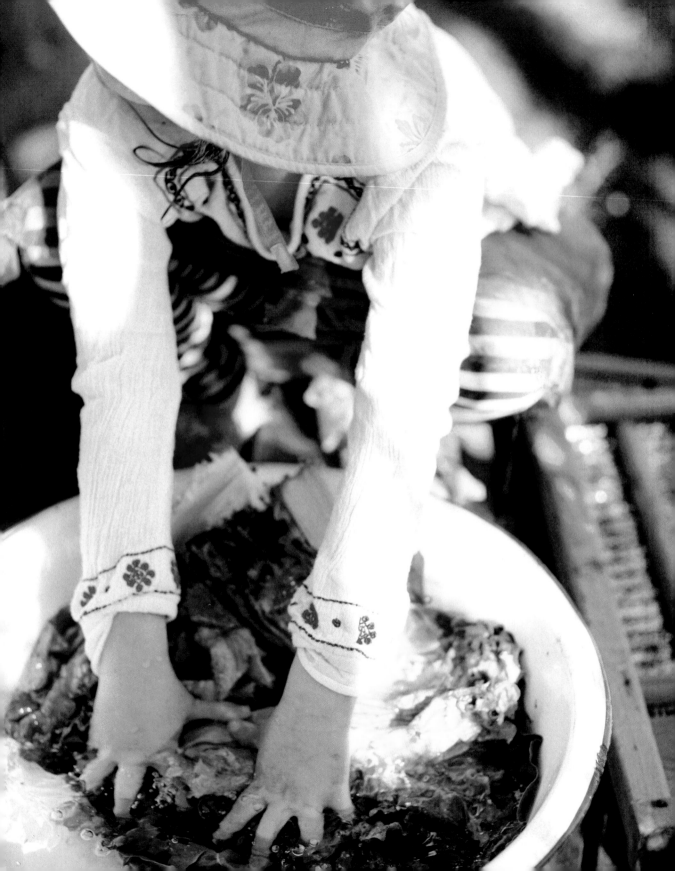

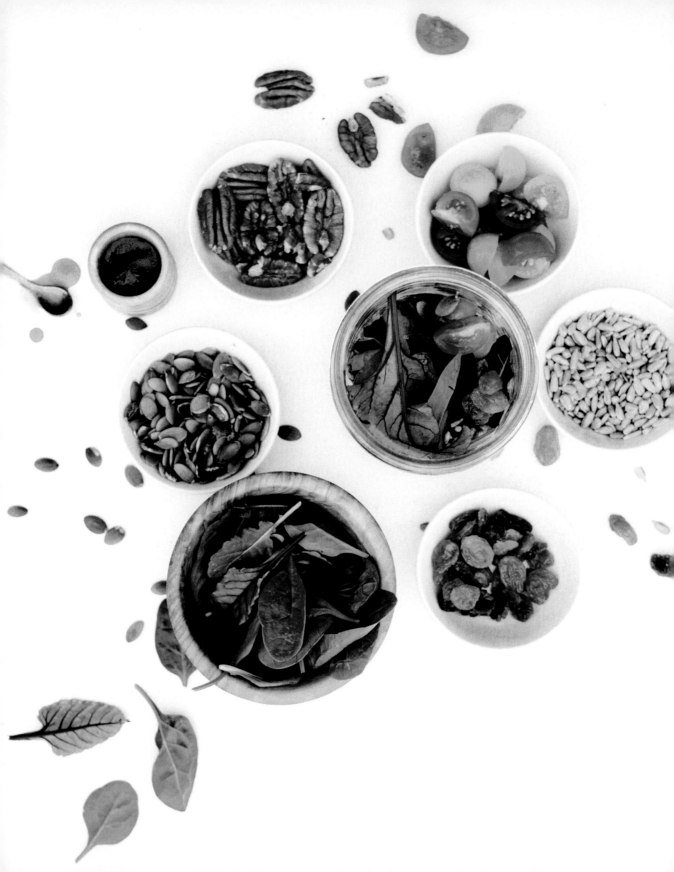

SALAD BAR IN A MASON JAR

SERVES 4

DRESSING

Choose from those on pages 137–140

GREENS (Choose 2)

I cup spinach

I cup red or green leaf lettuce

I cup butter lettuce

I cup romaine

I cup kale

I cup pea shoots

VEGGIES AND FRUITS (Choose 2)

½ cup garbanzo beans

½ cup halved grapes

½ cup grated carrots

½ cup halved cherry tomatoes

½ cup grated red cabbage

½ cup sprouts

CRUNCHIES (Choose 2)

¼ cup sunflower seeds

¼ cup pumpkin seeds

¼ cup pecans

¼ cup slivered almonds

¼ cup croutons

¼ cup crispy wontons

¼ cup Parmesan shavings

One way to invite even the most skeptical salad eater into the joy of salad is to celebrate the power of choice. This build-a-salad in a jar gives kids control. We like to set up the salad toppings in individual ramekins and line them up as a salad bar. Then we give each kid an eight-ounce mason jar and let them go wild and fill the jars with whatever they wish. Bonus: kids get to shake those little salad jars to distribute the dressing. What follows is a list of ingredients we love in our salad jars: choose as many as make sense for your own salad bar, but be sure to include at least some ingredients that your kid has already accepted instead of exclusively unfamiliar or not-yet-accepted ingredients.

Kid's job! Prep the veggies. Give them a cool bath, then pat dry with paper towels. Get your grating claw on (page 33). Now get grating and chopping.

Start building your salad-bar jar by picking an item or items from each section and get layering.

Dressing first. When building your salad bar in a mason jar, always start with the dressing. Pour 1 or 2 tablespoons of your favorite salad dressing or vinaigrette into the bottom of your jar.

A perfect foundation. You want the first layer to maintain its shape while mingling with, even marinating in, the dressing for a little while. This means sturdy veggies and legumes: beans, carrots, and the like. This layer also prevents the greens from getting soggy while hanging out in the fridge overnight, in your lunch box during the school day, or in your backpack while you take a hike.

Layer it up. Load up on your greens, then add anything light, crunchy, or cheesy.

Be sure to leave a little empty space at the top of your jar for shaking room, then screw your lid on tightly. When it's time to eat, give your jar the shake of its life.

LET US DO A LETTUCE TASTE TEST

SOME LETTUCES

Romaine: crunchy and mild

Red-leaf romaine: sweet and crunchy

Butter: velvety yum

Baby spinach: super tender and mild

Arugula (the Brits call this "rocket"): peppery bite

Frisée: frizzy texture

Kale: bitter

Radicchio: bitter and crunchy

Do you know there are so many different types of lettuce that you could eat a different kind every day for almost a year? Each variety looks—and tastes—different. West will snub an entire salad upon detecting a single leaf of arugula ("too spicy"), but he'll devour an unreasonably large trough of baby spinach in one sitting. If your kid thinks she doesn't like salad greens, we challenge you to do a lettuce taste test. While you're at it, throw in some other leafy greens. When we were kids, grocery stores pretty much offered only iceberg and romaine. Today, many stores offer an assortment of salad vegetables from purple radicchio to ten kinds of kale. We firmly believe there's a leafy green out there for every kid and every grown-up. Start the quest to find your family's favorite greens.

KIDS ▶ CHOOSE LEAFY VEGGIES

Go to your grocery store. How many different types of lettuce are available? We've listed some lettuces you might find, so pick two or three you've never tasted.

MAKE A LETTUCE PLATTER

When you get home, wash and dry your lettuces. Put one leaf of each kind of lettuce on a plate. Set up three of your favorite dressings to dip your leaves into. Taste each one.

Record Your Findings:

Today, our family tried these new lettuces:

The lettuce with the loudest crunch:

Sweetest lettuce:

The lettuce that makes the best hat:

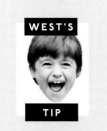

WEST'S

TIP

Freeze fresh baby spinach leaves and eat them like chips straight out of the freezer.

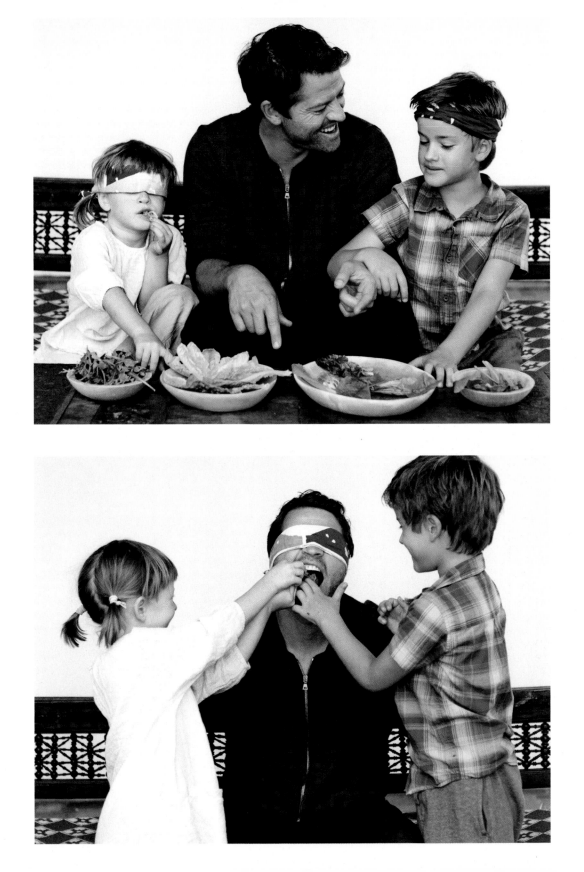

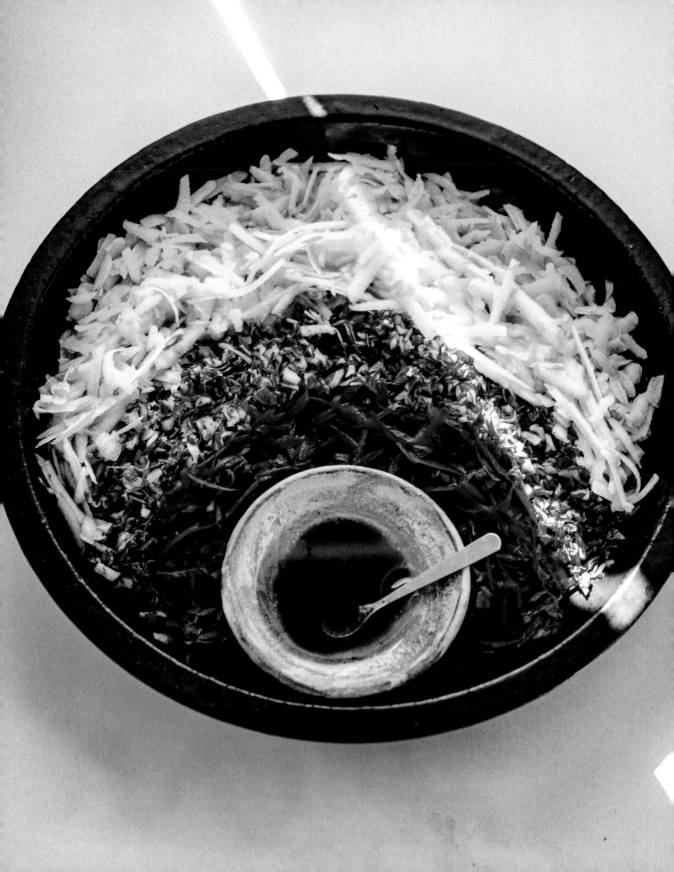

HALF-RAINBOW SLAW

SERVES 4

1 cup grated raw beets

1 cup grated carrots

1 cup thinly sliced
red cabbage

1 cup grated apple
(Granny Smith)

2 tablespoons olive oil

1 tablespoon balsamic
vinegar

Sea salt to taste

Raisins (optional)

Sesame seeds
(optional)

This flashy colorful slaw was the first salad West fell in love with, and it remains one of his favorites. With its tart flavor and satisfying crunch, it turned West into such a die-hard cabbage lover that he's now determined to invent a cabbage-flavored cotton candy. (Don't worry: we haven't gone there . . . yet.) Let your kids do all the grating so they get the chance to work with these colorful veggies.

Kid's job! Grate, grate, and grate some more! Use the regular large grater holes to grate the carrots, beets, and apple. Use the gigantic slicer hole on the grater to grate the red cabbage.

In a separate bowl, whisk together olive oil and balsamic vinegar. Add salt.

Serve each element separately with a little bowl of dressing on the side so kids can pick and choose which stripe in the rainbow to taste.

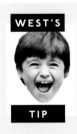

WEST'S

TIP

How about sprinkling something crunchy on top? How about salty roasted sunflower seeds? Crushed peanuts? Crushed corn chips? You decide.

SWEET CORN SUMMER SALAD

SERVES 4 TO 6

3 ears fresh sweet corn

1 pint cherry tomatoes, halved

⅓ cup olive oil

Juice of 1 lemon

Sea salt to taste

There is nothing more naturally delicious than sweet summer corn, and this salad celebrates that flavor perfectly. If you've got a yard and a picnic table, you're going to want to start making this salad out there, because the mess potential for corn shucking is off the charts. Give the kids a couple of ears to shuck while you start on the parts of the meal that involve advanced knife skills.

Kid's job! Shuck the corn. Over the sink, on your porch, wherever it may be, start peeling away the thick green outer husk. Then yank those silky strings from each cob. Can you make a skirt or a hat from the corn husks?

In a large pot, bring about two inches of water to a boil. Place the corn in the pot stem ends down. Cover and steam for about 8 to 10 minutes. Using tongs, remove the corn from the water. Dunk the corn into a big bowl of cold water.

Once the corn is cool enough to handle, slice the tip off each ear to create a flat surface. Resting the flat surface of the ear on a cutting board, hold the stem end with one hand while using a sharp knife to saw off the kernels in a downward motion, rotating the ear to get every last sweet golden corn nugget.

Combine the kernels and tomatoes in a large bowl. Drizzle with olive oil and lemon juice, and season with salt. Stir and enjoy the crunchy sweetness of this fresh and summery corn creation.

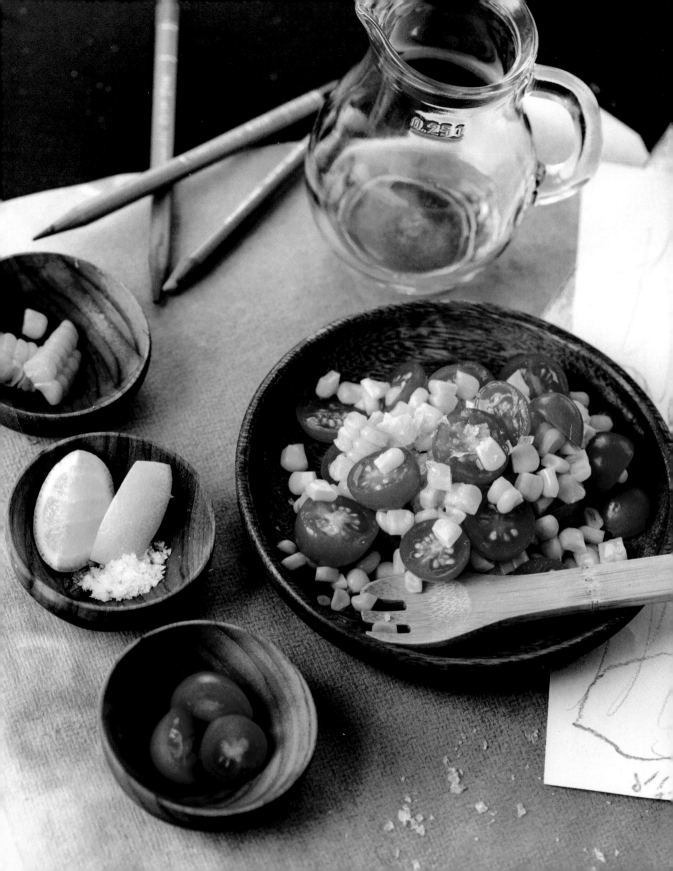

KALE, KALE

AND MORE KALE

One of the most effective ways to welcome hesitant eaters to the wonders of salad is to use just two or three ingredients and a simple dressing. In our family, our go-to salad has only five ingredients: kale (we like to use dino kale, but any kale works), Parmesan cheese, lemon juice, olive oil, and sea salt. Our whole family has fallen for this simple salad. West and Maison make the entire salad themselves, adjusting proportions as they taste along the way.

Kid's job! First wash the kale. Then destem it. Grab on to the "handle" of the stem with one hand, and use the other hand to tear the leaves away in one sweeping motion. Scream *"Hi-ya!"* as you rip the leaves off. Then tear up the leaves.

Throw them in the salad spinner. Spin until completely dry.

Toss the dried torn leaves into a big bowl, squeeze a lemon wedge over them, and add a big pinch of sea salt.

Using clean hands, squeeze, squish, and massage the leaves until they turn a dark green and soften. Put some muscle into that massage! Keep going for a minute or two. Kale also loves to be serenaded. Is there a special song you've been itching to sing to your leafy greens? Belt it out. Once the kale has relaxed from its massage, add a little olive oil. Grate some Parm on top. Mix it up with your hands. Taste. What does it need to be tastier? You decide.

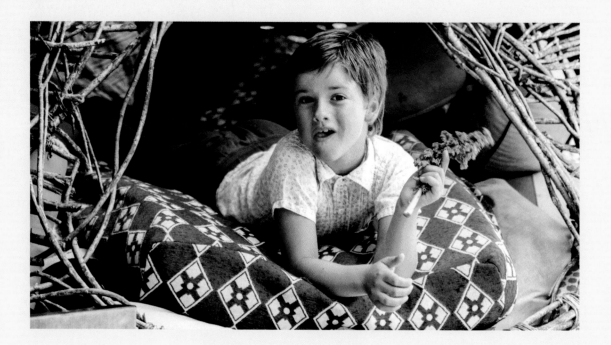

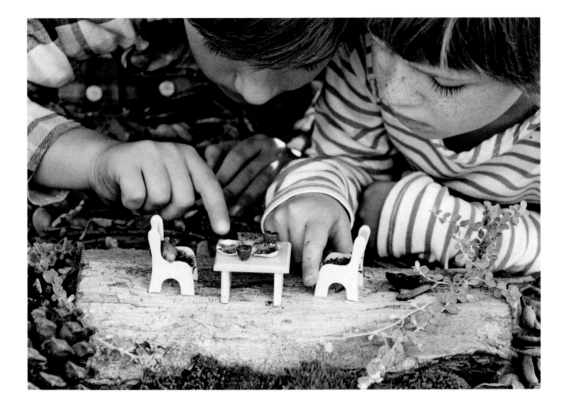

TURN YOUR KID
INTO A SALAD LOVER

Make a Fairy-Size Salad

Miniaturizing portions is a valuable strategy for introducing children to new foods, because minuscule portions are more approachable and less overwhelming, according to pediatric food experts. Is your kid freaked out by the prospect of eating an entire lettuce leaf? Invite her to make a Lilliputian salad inside a thimble. Sometimes Maison uses tweezers to lay a microscopic carrot shaving on top of her "elf salad." She eats the entire thing in one bite.

BREAD SALAD

SERVES 3 TO 4

4 to 5 cups 2-inch bread chunks (about 8 ounces) from baguettes or any hearty, crusty artisan bread

¼ cup olive oil

Sea salt to taste

1 head romaine lettuce, leaves torn

1 to 3 large tomatoes (get the in-season, juicy heirloom ones if possible), roughly chopped

¾ cup shaved Parmesan cheese

DRESSING

¼ cup olive oil

2 tablespoons red wine vinegar

Sea salt to taste

Most American children are pretty familiar with bread. We've found that a nice crusty loaf makes a fun bridge to salad for kids beginning to explore salads. This recipe also involves making your own croutons, which is fun for kids. West tends to pick the bread out and eat only the veggies. One of his best friends eats only the bread. This recipe is most glorious in the summer, when tomatoes are at their prime.

Preheat the oven to 350°F.

To make the croutons, spread the bread chunks on a sheet pan and drizzle with olive oil. Sprinkle with salt, then toss to coat. Bake for about 15 minutes, stirring once or twice during the cooking, until the chunks are slightly hard and starting to color.

Kid's job! Put the chunks in a zip-lock bag. Squeeze the extra air out before you zip the bag closed. Using a wooden mallet or the bottom of a heavy pan, give the toasted chunks a few good whacks to break your croutons into smaller bites.

To make the dressing, whisk together the olive oil, vinegar, and salt in a large salad bowl.

Add the bread, lettuce, tomatoes, and Parm. Use a spatula to thoroughly mix, so all the bread is coated in the dressing and the juice from the tomatoes.

This is the tricky part. Let the salad rest at room temperature (don't refrigerate) for at least 30 minutes, so all the juices soak into the bread and mingle. Give the salad a stir a few times. Serve when the dressing is thoroughly soaked into the bread.

THE YOUNG BOTANIST'S TOMATO TEST

Some children don't take to tomatoes right away. First things first: not all tomatoes are created equal. Beware the winter tomato. Few off-season veggies are as disappointing as this mealy, watery, tasteless beast. Would you like tomatoes if a December beefsteak was all you had to judge by? If your kids aren't tomato fiends yet, wait until these fruits are in season. Make a game out of letting your child pick five different varieties of the brightly colored ripe beauties from your local grocery store or farmers' market for a tomato taste test.

3 to 5 Sun Gold cherry tomatoes (these are so sweet we call them candy tomatoes)

1 to 2 heirloom tomatoes

3 to 5 red cherry tomatoes

1 orange tomato

1 yellow tomato

1 Roma (plum) tomato

2 tablespoons olive oil

2 tablespoons balsamic vinegar

2 tablespoons sea salt

2 tablespoons chopped fresh basil

2 tablespoons grated Parmesan cheese

Set up a tomato tasting station. Wash and dry your tomatoes. Quarter the cherry tomatoes. Slice other tomatoes into ¼-inch slices. Arrange them on a plate to make a rainbow of tomatoes to taste.

Set out tiny dishes filled with olive oil, balsamic vinegar, sea salt, basil, and grated Parm. Let the kids choose how to dress each tomato slice.

Name your favorite dressed tom-tom.
What did you put on top?

SLIPPERY AND CRUNCHY, SWEET AND SALTY SUPER SPRING SALAD

SERVES 4 TO 6

2 tablespoons
maple syrup

½ cup walnut halves

Sea salt to taste

15 seedless grapes,
or more to taste

2 heaping cups
mixed greens

1 tablespoon
walnut oil

Our kids love this salad, and we suspect yours will, too. This is an unusual salad because it doesn't have any acidic elements. No lemon, no vinegar. So it really lets the flavors of the simple ingredients pop in your mouth.

MISHA SAYS: When I graduated from college, my roommate took me out to a fancy restaurant in Chicago as a graduation present. It was the most elegant place I'd ever been to. It had only four tables. They served a salad with peeled grapes and candied walnuts. I was head over heels, and I've been re-creating that salad ever since. This is our family's version.

Line a sheet pan with parchment paper and set aside.

Warm the maple syrup in a small skillet over medium heat. Add walnuts and salt. Stir the syrup with a spatula until it becomes caramelly and gooey, about 3 minutes. Scrape the nuts out onto the parchment-lined sheet pan and spread them into a single layer. Let cool. Once cool, the walnuts will harden like candy.

Kid's job! Some of the nuts will stick together. Once they are cooled, break them apart.

Kid's job! Peel the grapes. Here's where focus and concentration come in handy. Can you peel the skin off a grape? Yes, it requires the concentration of an Olympic skier and the nimbleness of a surgeon. You've got this. Peel some grapes. If you do 5, great. If you can do 10, even better. If you're really keen on mastering your grape-peeling skills, go for 15. Now slice each grape in half. Set aside. Taste one. Does it taste yummier than an unpeeled grape? We think so.

In a large salad or mixing bowl, combine the greens with the walnut oil. Add the grapes and candied nuts. Toss, salt to taste, and toss again. Serve.

ELF LEAF SALAD

SERVES 4 TO 6

2 cups destemmed kale leaves (page 126)

9 to 10 ounces brussels sprouts

Generous pinch of sea salt

2-ounce block Parmesan cheese

¼ cup sliced almonds

¼ cup raisins

DRESSING

1 tablespoon balsamic vinegar

3 tablespoons olive oil

½ tablespoon maple syrup

Generous pinch of sea salt

Brussels sprouts are notoriously icky for kids (and many adults). But served raw as elfin leaves, and covered in a juicy dressing, they offer an entirely new and delicious eating experience.

Thinly slice the kale.

Kid's job! Pull the leaves off of the brussels sprouts, leaving the inner core behind. You should have about 3 cups of leaves. Throw the leaves into the big bowl with the kale. Add the salt, then give the greens a relaxing massage.

Kid's job! Using a grizzly-claw hand (page 33), grip your block of Parm and grate it on the large holes of a box grater. Set aside.

Toast the almonds in a small dry saucepan over medium heat. Stir for 3 to 5 minutes, until lightly golden. Taste. Set aside.

To make the dressing, combine the vinegar, olive oil, maple syrup, and salt in a small bowl and whisk. Taste and adjust the seasoning as needed.

Add the toasted almonds and raisins to the bowl of shredded kale and sprout leaves. Pour a little dressing over the greens, toss, add the Parm, and toss again. Taste. Add more dressing if you like. Serve.

RAISIN TASTE TEST

This salad provides a perfect opportunity to test Misha's personal theory that raisins make every dish more delicious. Our family is deeply divided on this issue. (Vicki is a firm believer that raisins do not make every dish tastier. Consider clam chowder with and without raisins, if you will.) Put half the salad in one bowl and the other half in another bowl. Add raisins to the first half. Taste the salad in both bowls. Do raisins make this salad more delicious? Yes/No. Vote.

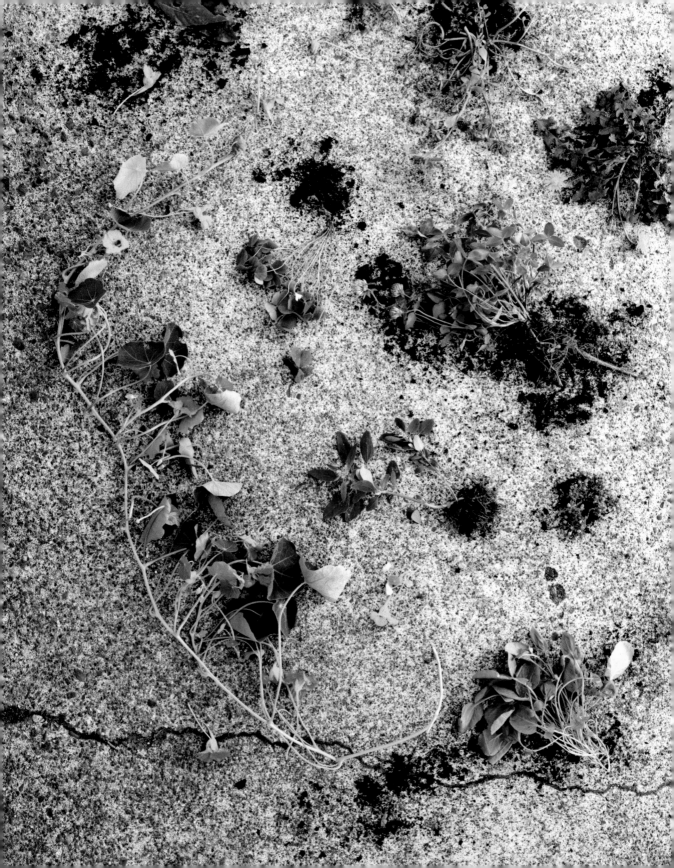

Adventure Recipe
SIDEWALK CRACK SALAD

There's a good chance that there's a smorgasbord of salad greens growing in your own backyard or in nearby sidewalk cracks. Many common weeds are surprisingly tasty—and they're totally free. Here are some common North American edible wild plants that make a tasty salad.

Dandelion: Familiar weed with edible yellow blossoms and leaves

Purslane: Succulent with reddish stems with a slightly lemony taste

Watercress: Expensive grocery-store go-to weed that grows along streambeds in nearly every state

Red clover: Edible pink blossoms

Wood sorrel: Shamrock-shaped leaves and tiny blossoms with a lemony burst of flavor

Lamb's quarters: Tastes like a cross between spinach and Swiss chard

Nasturtium: Large bright orange or yellow flowers on a common vine with a peppery punch

Pineapple weed: Fruity-flavored edible found in fields, playgrounds, and yards nationwide; crush the flower for a pineapple scent

Take your kids for a stroll around your backyard or neighborhood. Which edible weeds can you find? Gather your harvested flowers and greens and give them a good wash in cold water. Now pat them dry with a towel or put them in the salad spinner. Throw them all into a big salad bowl and add your favorite dressing.

Notes on foraging: Triple-confirm that you've identified a plant properly before consuming it. (There are poisonous plants out there, for goodness' sake.) There are plenty of foraging guidebooks on the market as well as plant-identification apps (like Wild Edibles) that can help. If you're really jazzed about finding edibles in your 'hood, take a tour with a local foraging expert such as Steve Brill, a botanist known for his edible-plant tours of New York City's Central Park.

Steer clear of areas that may have been treated with pesticides or chemicals. If you're harvesting near your neighbors' lawns, ask them if they use pesticides, since you'll want to avoid weeds near sprayed areas. Check with city hall or park officials to find out if pesticides are used in public areas. Avoid areas with a lot of pet traffic.

Make sure your kids know that they need a grown-up's confirmation that a wild plant is edible before they eat it.

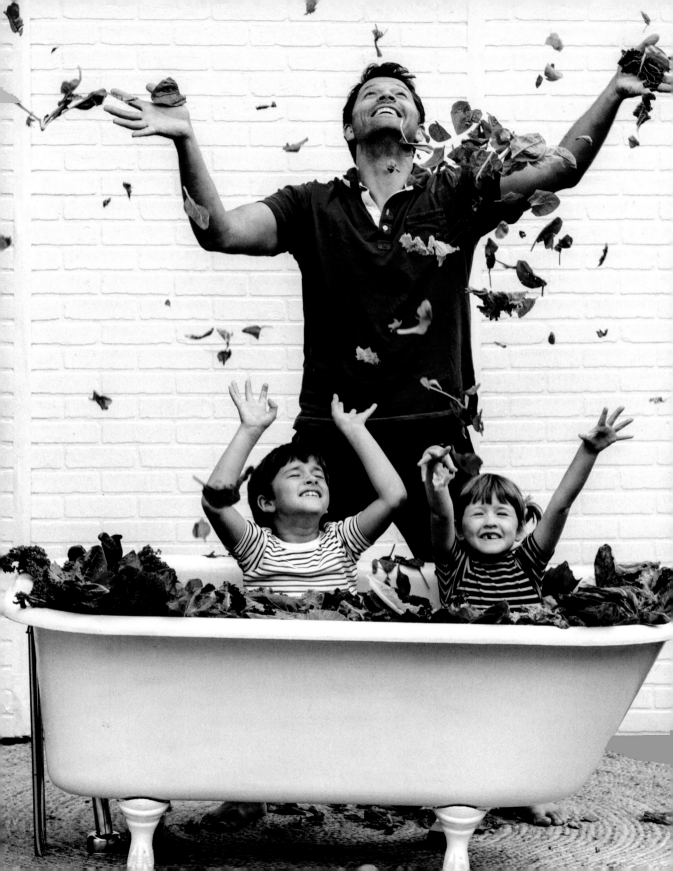

Culinary Frontiers

West's Santa Monica Winter Salad

1 red cabbage

1 green cabbage

1 Chinese cabbage

1 head iceberg lettuce

Handful of peanuts in shells

1 can corn chowder

Skin of 1 red onion

Prepackaged turkey gravy for serving

West invented this salad at age three, during an episode of *Cooking Fast & Fresh with West*. It's absolutely not recommended—for kids or adults.

Chop the cabbages and lettuce and combine them in a large salad bowl. Add peanuts (in shells). Pour the can of cold corn chowder over the salad as dressing. Garnish with onion skin. Serve this with a side of gravy. Enjoy.

Or, you know . . . don't.

SALAD DRESSINGS

Dressing can play an important role in converting resistant children into salad enthusiasts. Contrary to popular belief, that doesn't mean you need to smother salad in ketchup or ranch dressing to make it edible to young 'uns. Let your kids be in charge of making the dressing. Let them taste and adjust it for their own palate. Some kids prefer an acidic dressing; others like more sweetness or more oil. Letting them play a part in making their food makes them more likely to eat it.

WEST'S GO-TO DRESSING

MAKES ½ CUP

¼ cup balsamic vinegar

½ teaspoon honey

¼ cup olive oil

Sea salt to taste

Combine the balsamic vinegar and honey in a small jar with a tight-fitting lid. Screw on the lid and shake vigorously for a few seconds—this preliminary shake will help the dressing blend well. Add the oil and salt and give it another good shake. Taste. What does it need more of?

Store in the fridge for up to ten days, and give it a good shake before each use.

VINAIGRETTE

MAKES ½ CUP

½ shallot, minced

2 tablespoons red wine vinegar

Sea salt to taste

6 tablespoons olive oil

Combine the shallot, vinegar, and salt in a small bowl. Let the mixture sit for 15 minutes, then add the olive oil and whisk to emulsify.

Store in the fridge for up to ten days, and give it a good shake before each use.

JUICE DRESSING

MAKES ¼ CUP

2 tablespoons freshly squeezed lemon juice

2 tablespoons olive oil

½ teaspoon honey

Sea salt to taste

Combine the lemon juice and honey in a small jar with a tight-fitting lid. Screw on the lid and shake vigorously for a few seconds. Add the oil and salt and give it another good shake. Taste.

Store in the fridge for up to ten days, and give it a good shake before each use.

THE "STRAWBERRIES ARE GOOD" DRESSING

Maison invented (and named) this dressing, which we love. It's the first salad dressing our five-year-old neighbor has ever tasted and liked. (Of course, he still hasn't actually dipped a piece of lettuce in it, but that's a technicality.)

MAKES ABOUT 1 CUP

1 cup roughly chopped fresh strawberries, stems removed

2 tablespoons freshly squeezed lime juice

1 tablespoon balsamic vinegar

¼ cup olive oil

1 teaspoon honey

Sea salt to taste

Combine all ingredients in a blender. Add 1 tablespoon water and zip the ingredients for a few seconds, until smooth. Pour the pink dressing over your favorite salad or slaw. Maison would say this dressing goes great on every salad; it lasts a few days in the refrigerator.

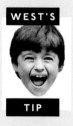

WEST'S TIP

HOW TO DRESS A SALAD: Once you've masterminded your own dressing, get ready to dress the salad. Wash and dry the leaves. Get them really dry! Dressing sticks to dry leaves better. Pluck out any wilted or yucky leaves. No one likes a limp leaf! Throw your dried lettuce into a big bowl. Go big so you can get your hands in there. Add some dressing. Use one hand to toss the leaves around so they get coated. I like a LOT of balsamic vinegar in my dressing. Maison likes it really salty. How do YOU like it? Taste. What would make it yummier? More salt? More lemon? Maple syrup? You decide! Now make that salad pretty. Add some purple rosemary flowers on top. Eat it right away—use chopsticks, tongs, or even your hands. You're allowed to use a fork, but why would you do that?!

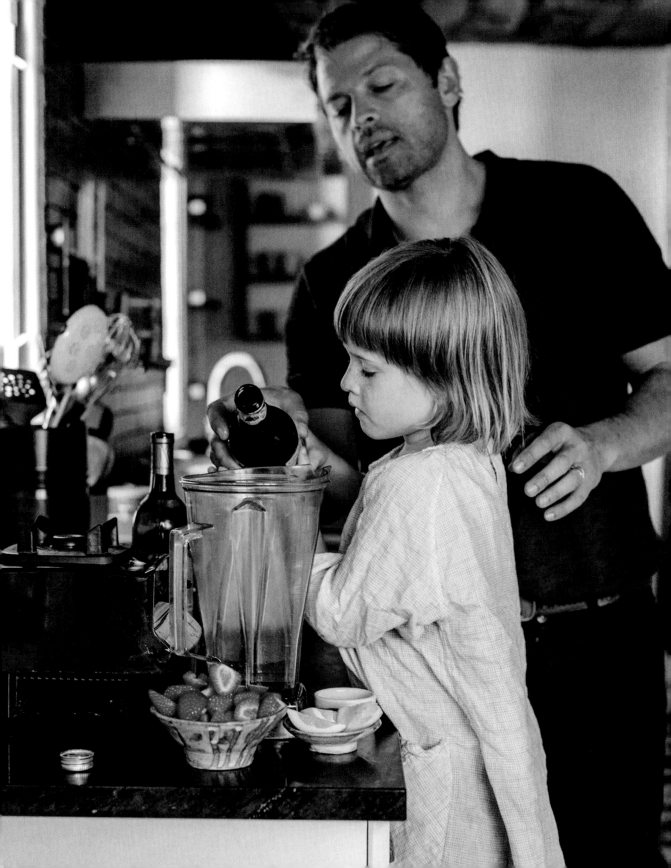

Adventure Recipe
TOMATO-SEED VINAIGRETTE

MAKES ½ TO 1 CUP, DEPENDING ON HOW JUICY YOUR TOM-TOMS ARE

1 pint cherry tomatoes

2 tablespoons freshly squeezed lemon juice

1 teaspoon honey

½ cup olive oil

Sea salt to taste

We've all had the line "Don't play with your food" drilled into our heads, but we encourage you to boldly ignore Emily Post and get down and dirty with it. Many young children are freaked out by tomatoes because of the unpredictable way they squirt. Playing with the fruit can help kids get comfortable with these seedy treats by desensitizing them to the squirt factor. Even if your kid doesn't taste this dressing, the process of making it can help tomato-shy kids get one step closer to biting into one. Set this adventure recipe up outside, or you'll be scraping rogue seeds off your ceiling for months.

Kid's job! Squirt the seeds. Set up a large, wide-rimmed bowl a few inches away from your tomatoes. Put on goggles if you like. Now use your fingers to pop and squirt the seeds from your teeny tomatoes. Hold a tomato between your thumb and your forefinger, give it a good squeeze, and watch the seeds fly. Can you aim them into the bowl? Are some tomatoes juicier than others? There's only one way to find out—give them a good squeeze and watch them squirt. Feel free to taste the skins as you go, since we only want the seeds and juice for this dressing.

Now that you have a bowl full of juicy tomato innards, add the lemon juice and honey to the bowl. Whisk, then drizzle in the olive oil and salt.

FAMILY CHALLENGE

KID CHEF IN CHARGE

What happens when parents embrace the wonder (and horror) of freestyle cooking with a kid at the helm? We decided to find out. When West was two years old, we performed an experiment. We set him loose in a grocery store and let him prepare dinner with all the ingredients he selected. The results were . . . unconventional. A gustatory madman, West invented some intriguing (and undeniably inedible) dishes, including his signature Pasta with Jam Sauce (page 172), which features boiled chocolate chips, a half-eaten apple, Goldfish, and pasta.

We challenge you to reverse roles with your kid. Let him be the head chef for one meal. He gets to buy the ingredients and cook them however he wishes. We dare you . . .

Step 1: The Shopping Trip

Give your kids a few parameters and a budget for a trip to the grocery store. Perhaps they can purchase anything from the fresh produce section, any meat, any dairy. Perhaps they're limited to purchasing only one small sweet to serve for dessert so that you don't end up eating a mountain of gummy bears stuffed into a watermelon (trust us, this can happen when you set a child free in a grocery store).

Step 2: Cooking It Up Their Way

Once shopping is done, your kid gets to be the head chef—and make dinner her way. Your job, parents, is to say "yes, *and*" to your kid's culinary vision for the meal, whatever it is. She wants to use the hand mixer to whip dry pasta into a bowl of orange juice? Absolutely. Flipping the script on who's in charge can be really liberating. It can inspire kids to create new flavor combinations and feel empowered in the kitchen.

Warning: Letting your kid lead in the kitchen requires some serious letting go. Unexpected flavor combinations may occur. Do not try this at home if you don't have several hours to clean up or if the thought of mixing savory with sweet gives you hives. Exactly zero pediatric dietitians recommend this strategy. We only cook this way on special occasions—and we are known for engaging in totally unreasonable, ill-advised activities.

Jot down your kid's culinary creations.

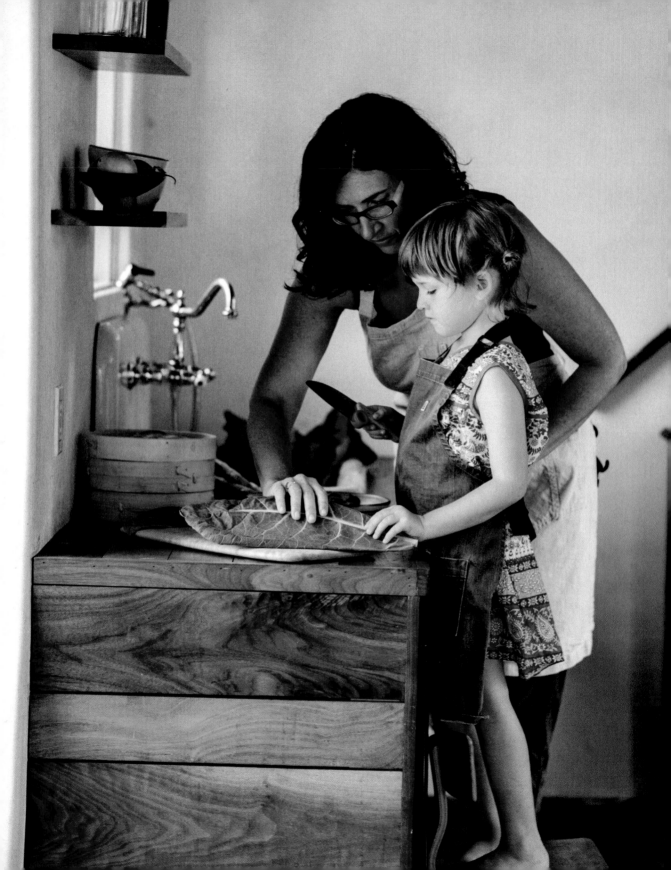

MAINS

Most of the meals we included in this chapter are fast (thirty minutes or less) and healthful, sure, but what we really love about these recipes is that they offer a portal to food-loving adventures for burgeoning young chefs. Our family developed many of these recipes by improvising together in the kitchen—experimenting with unfamiliar spices, attempting to boil cantaloupe, and laughing . . . a lot. We chose recipes that we love making together, and we hope they inspire your family to find adventure in your kitchen and at your table.

ADVENTUROUS KID EATERS SAY...

MILES, AGE SIX

Food I didn't used to like that I like now: Bananas.

I like to eat: Yams, sushi, vanilla beans, grilled salmon, french fries, kale, green beans, chives, raspberries, meat sticks, seaweed, and broccoli.

If I had my own restaurant, I'd call it: Eeny Meeny Miney Steak.

Weirdest thing I've ever tasted: Squid! I was four years old when I tried it. I liked it, but it was really weird—maybe because I tried it with a noodle dipped in chocolate sauce. Not sure.

My idea for a new recipe that I think I'd love: Chocolate-flavored chili soup.

MISHA'S TAKE ON FAMILY DINNER: I won't lecture you about the value of eating home-cooked family dinners. Rumor has it that family dinner is a good thing. In my fantasy version of myself, I'm home every night, dicing garden-fresh carrots, snipping herbs in the garden, and preparing a beautiful dinner. I should also mention that this version of me is totally present, relaxed, and *extremely* fun. This version of me is not feeling at all overwhelmed by the stuff I was supposed to do but haven't or the unconscionable volume of emails waiting in my in-box. This me is a stellar dad who has plenty of time to plant a garden with my kids, bake Pinterest-perfect casseroles, and whittle wooden tops. Needless to say, the gulf between the fantasy me and the real-world me is wide, but even when I'm busy and overworked, if I can find time to cook, I know I haven't gone completely off the rails. Cooking grounds me and helps take my mind off the chatter of the outside world. When I'm in the kitchen making dinner with West and Maison, it feels like all is well.

WISHING WELL SOUP

SERVES 4 TO 6

I boneless, skinless chicken breast, about 6 ounces

Sea salt to taste

I cup dried alphabet pasta

I tablespoon butter

2 carrots, chopped

2 celery stalks, chopped

¼ cup minced red onion

6 cups chicken broth

2 bay leaves

2 large lacinato, or dino, kale leaves, destemmed and thinly sliced

In the winter, we always have a big pot of soup on our stove. We like experimenting with a new soup each week. Soup begs for improvisation—so we let our kids ad-lib. Plus, it's quick and easy to warm up for lunches. West likes to try to eat a whole bowl of it without a spoon by dunking and redunking a buttery piece of toast. In our home, we love hearty options—this one is simple and brimming with veggies and secret wishes.

Season the chicken breast with salt. Cut it up into tiny chunks and set aside.

Meanwhile, bring a pot of water to boil and cook the pasta according to package directions. Drain and set aside.

In a medium pot, melt the butter over medium heat. Add the chicken and sauté for a minute or so, then add the carrot, celery, and onion. Cook, stirring frequently, for 4 to 5 minutes, or until the veggies are tender and the onion is translucent.

Add the broth and bay leaves, stir, and bring to a boil. Lower the heat, then simmer until the chicken is cooked through and the veggies are tender, about 8 to 10 minutes. Adjust the seasoning as desired.

Remove the pot from the heat, then add the kale and alphabet pasta. Taste, adjust seasoning, and taste again. Serve. Whoever finds a bay leaf in his or her bowl gets to make a wish. (Don't eat the bay leaf—just wish on it.)

STEAMED GREEN DUMPLINGS

**MAKES 10
DUMPLINGS**

DUMPLINGS

½ pound ground beef

¼ teaspoon grated
fresh ginger

I teaspoon finely
chopped scallions
(white and tender green
parts only)

½ tablespoon soy sauce

½ tablespoon ketchup

¼ teaspoon sea salt

10 small collard leaves
(from about 2 bunches)

DIPPING SAUCE

½ clove garlic, minced
(about ¼ teaspoon)

¼ teaspoon grated
fresh ginger

I teaspoon finely
chopped scallion

I tablespoon raspberry
jam

2 tablespoons
sesame oil

2 tablespoons rice
vinegar

I tablespoon
soy sauce

Every culture in the world seems to have some form of dumpling it embraces as its own. From Polish pierogi to Italian ravioli to Taiwanese soup dumplings, the world loves a little dough pocket stuffed with goodness. When Misha was a kid, his best friend's family used to make Tibetan dumplings called momos, which he'd devour. Decades later, they're still Misha's comfort food. "During my first year away at college, I was homesick, and I asked my childhood best friend to make them for my birthday. Just the smell of these dumplings will make you feel better, I promise," says Misha. As a family, we've adapted the recipe by using steamed greens for the wrappers instead of dough. The dumplings' Asian taste may be new to some kids in the US, so we added a touch of ketchup to construct a familiar flavor bridge. West reports: "This smells like salty Chinese soup!" Maison says, "I love it." If the leafy wrappers are too much of a leap for your family, try using premade wonton wrappers, sold at most grocery stores, instead of collard greens.

Bring a few inches of water to a boil in a pot equipped with a steamer basket and a tight-fitting lid. Keep the basket out of the pot—you'll be snuggling your dumplings into it before putting it over the boiling water.

Kid's job! Make the filling: combine the beef, ginger, scallion, soy sauce, ketchup, and salt in a large bowl. Use your hands to mash it all together. Then wash your hands *really* well.

Destem each collard leaf by first laying it flat, with the dark side down and the pale underside facing up. Then slice along both sides of the stem lengthwise, leaving the top of your collard attached. Remove and discard the stem. You will be left with an upside-down V. Now you are ready to fill. Cross the collard "legs" one over the other to close the V.

Kid's job! Assemble the dumplings. Place a spoonful of filling in the bottom one-third of your collard wrap. From the bottom up, fold the leaf over the filling, then tuck in the sides tightly and continue rolling until you've burrito'd your way up to the top.

Holding the dumplings together with your fingers, lift and place them into your steamer basket one at a time. Fit as many dumplings as you can into a single layer—pack them in to keep them snug and tight while steaming. Place your steamer basket into the pot over the boiling water and cover. Steam for 10 minutes. Take the pot off the heat and use tongs to remove the dumplings.

Meanwhile, make the dipping sauce by whisking all ingredients together in a small bowl. Dunk your dumplings and enjoy. Definitely a finger food.

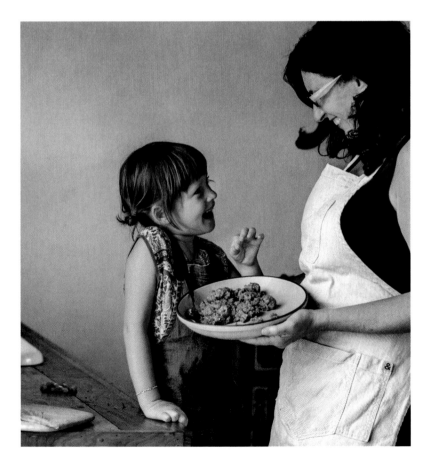

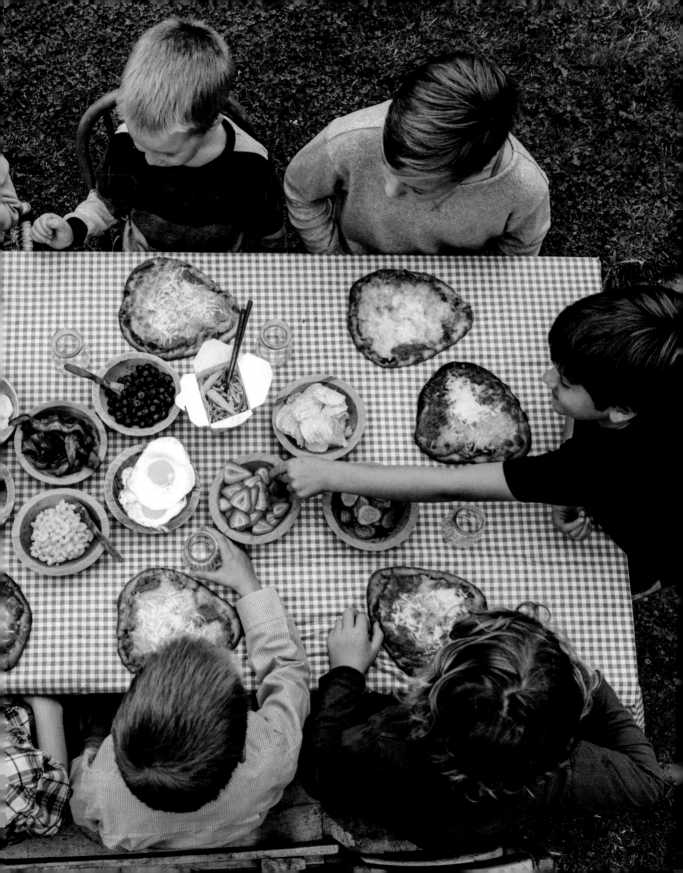

THE INVENTORS' PIZZA PARTY

**MAKES FOUR
5-INCH
PERSONAL PIZZAS**

BASE

Flour for dusting

I pound pizza dough

½ cup mild tomato sauce

A few kid-size fistfuls of shredded mozzarella cheese (about ¾ cup)

TOPPINGS

Shredded kale

Sliced strawberries

Scrambled eggs

Pickles

Mashed potatoes

Bananas

Bacon

Blueberries

Green beans

Mini pizzas on top of main pizza

Takeout leftovers

And anything else your children can think of!

We eat one hundred acres of pizza every day in the United States. That's three billion pizzas, or forty-six slices for every person, each year—topped with 251.7 million pounds of pepperoni. So it is no wonder most American kids are familiar with pizza. Learning to make it at home is one of the greatest kitchen adventures for budding chefs. Start with a classic margherita pizza and invite your young chefs to explore from there. You only need look as far as your kitchen—the fridge, the pantry: there's a world of possibilities there, including last night's leftovers. Our family relishes the challenge of making something that "no one has ever made before." Ask your kid what her dream 'za would be, then give it a shot. Bananas? Sure. Cereal? Well, okay. Let your kids get silly and choose ingredients that you'd normally veto. Encourage risky decisions. That's how genius culinary inventions come to pass, right? Maybe some of that kid creativity will even rub off on you and you'll invent a new pizza, too. Some combos will be, dare we say, unsuccessful (to say the least), but that's good news. Being creative and having fun in the kitchen are what we're after with this recipe.

Preheat the oven to 450°F. Pizza likes a really hot oven.

Kid's job! Work the dough. Give each person a sheet of parchment paper as a work surface. Sprinkle some flour on top of the paper. Each person gets a ball of dough the size of a hamster. Work the ball into a flat disk about one-quarter inch thick. Pick up the dough ball with both hands, then pinch and pull around and around the edges over and over until you have something resembling the beginnings of a pizza crust. Lay the dough disks back down onto the parchment and work them into squares, hearts, whatever you wish.

continued

Place your dough-topped pieces of parchment paper onto a cookie sheet. Top the dough with tomato sauce and shredded cheese. Bake for 10 to 15 minutes.

Kid's job! Put on your inventor's cap! While your pizzas are baking, daydream some toppings. For inspiration, check the canned foods in your pantry. Is there anything in there that might be tasty on pizza? Any fresh veggies that could really jazz it up? How about green bean pizza?

Set up your toppings station. Lay out a series of small bowls containing five different toppings you've never seen on pizza. We heartily recommend trying kale with strawberries.

Remove your pizzas from the oven. Now pile on the toppings. (If you suspect the toppings might be tastier warmed, throw the topped pizzas back in the oven for an additional minute or two.) Let the pizzas cool slightly, slice with a pizza cutter, and serve.

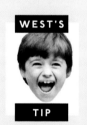

WEST'S TIP

I love fresh strawberries on pizza.

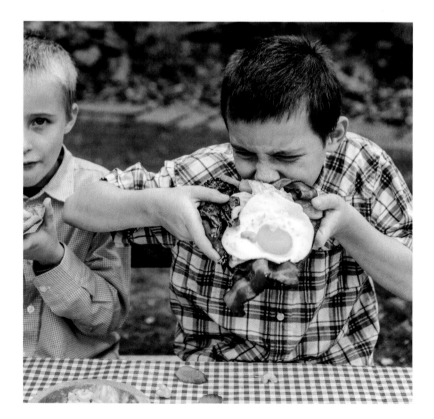

PANCAKES STUFFED WITH RAINBOWS

MAKES 6 PANCAKES

I cup all-purpose flour

¾ cup water

2 eggs

2 teaspoons soy sauce or tamari (for dipping)

Sea salt to taste

¼ cup kale ribbons (from I destemmed lacinato leaf)

½ cup shredded carrots

I cup grated red cabbage

4 to 6 teaspoons canola oil

We've been making some version of this pancake for years. These aren't the kind of pancakes that parents use to disguise veggies. These pancakes celebrate veggies—they're bursting with vibrant colors and crunch. We assumed these would be a definite no-go for Maison's best friend, who tends to favor peanut butter and Triscuits, so when we served these for dinner, we didn't put any on her plate. But she zeroed in on the pancake as soon as it landed and yanked it off Maison's plate. She wolfed it down and asked for another. We tried to conceal our glee, but this felt like a big win.

Mix the flour, water, egg, soy sauce, and salt in a large bowl until smooth. Stir in the kale, carrots, and cabbage.

Heat a small crepe or omelet pan over medium high heat. Swirl 1 teaspoon of oil in the pan, then pour in ¼ cup of the batter. Cook on one side until golden brown, 3 to 4 minutes. Flip. Cook on the other side for 2 to 3 minutes. Repeat until all the batter is used.

Salt to taste and serve with soy sauce for dipping.

PINK VEGGIE AND CHICKEN SPRING ROLLS

SERVES 4

¼ cup grated raw beets

¼ cup grated apple sprinkled with lemon juice (so it doesn't brown)

I cup cooked pulled chicken

Sea salt to taste

4 rice paper wrappers, or more if desired

DIPPING SAUCE

I tablespoon smooth peanut butter

I tablespoon soy sauce

I tablespoon freshly squeezed lime juice

I tablespoon sesame oil

I teaspoon honey

We love these simple fresh spring rolls. You can stuff nearly any ingredient inside, so let your kids follow their creative impulses when it comes to fillings. They work well packed in lunches, and the beets turn them neon pink.

Kid's job! To make the filling, combine your beets, apples, chicken, and salt in a big bowl. Use clean hands to mix. Taste. Does it need more salt? More apple? You decide.

Fill a shallow bowl or a pie pan with warm water. Carefully pick up a piece of rice paper with your hands—they're flimsy, so be gentle. Dip the paper into the water for a few seconds, until just soft. Lay the wet rice paper flat on a clean surface. Distribute a small spoonful of filling down the center of the paper, leaving all edges free.

Time to roll. Start with tucking in the top and bottom flaps of the paper over your line of filling. Now fold one side over the filling and, using your fingers, gently but tightly tuck and roll, as if you were making a burrito. The rice wrapper will be a little tacky and will self-seal all the filling in. Repeat with the remaining wrappers and filling. Lay the finished spring rolls on a plate lined with wet paper towels. Keep them from touching so they do not stick together.

To make the sauce, whisk all ingredients in a small bowl. Use 1 to 2 tablespoons water to thin the sauce to the desired consistency. Divide among four individual dipping bowls and serve.

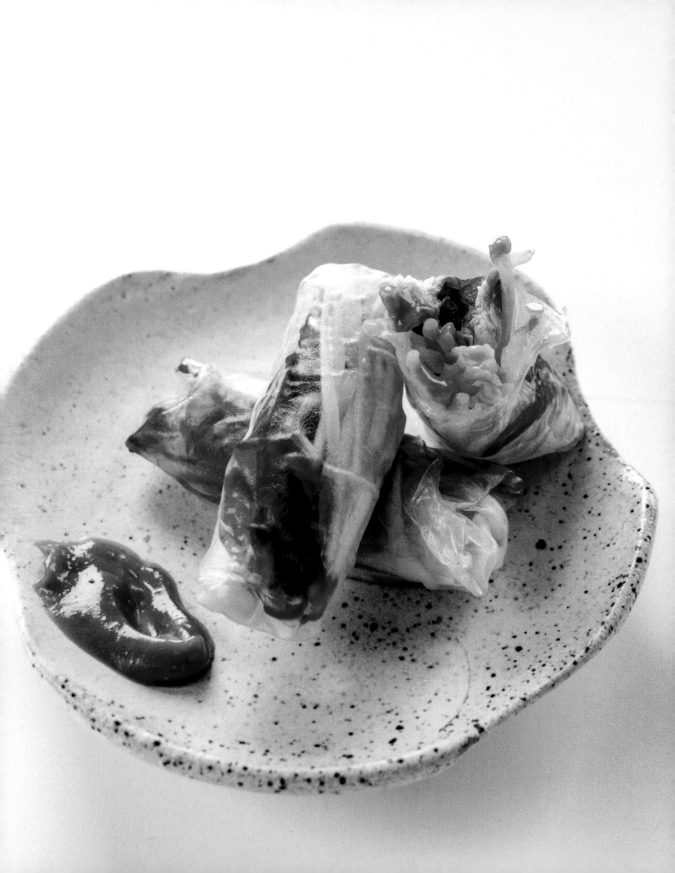

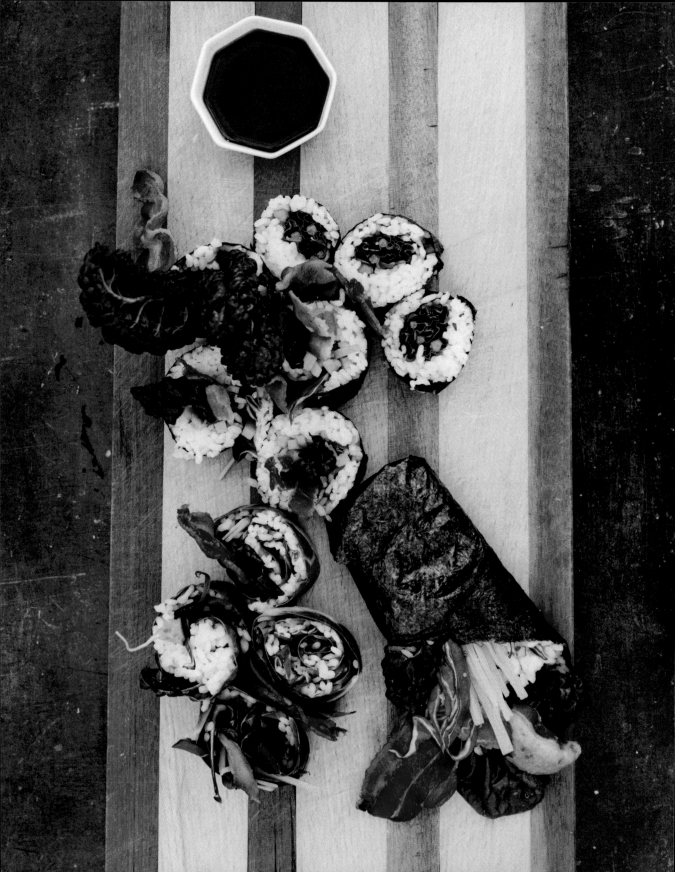

KALE AND BACON SUSHI

**MAKES 2
HAND ROLLS**

I cup sushi rice

2 strips bacon

2 nori (seaweed) sheets

2 leaves kale, destemmed
and thinly sliced

Soy sauce for dipping

As much as we love sashimi, our kids haven't gotten into raw fish yet, so we're starting slow by creating our own veggie—or veggie and meat—sushi rolls at home. This is West's favorite sushi invention and an inspirational template for devising your own combinations. Kids love making sushi because they can control what goes inside. Let them put in whatever they want—no matter how heretical. A bamboo mat makes this recipe easier to prep but isn't necessary.

Preheat the oven to 375°F.

Use a strainer to rinse uncooked rice until water runs clear. Cook the rice according to the package directions. We like to throw ours in the rice cooker. There are about a thousand different ways to cook rice; we aren't fussy. The goal is to have rice that stays starchy so that when you squeeze a handful it's quite sticky, which is best for sushi rolls.

Meanwhile, place the bacon on a tin-foil-lined baking sheet and bake for 15 minutes (or more if you like extra-crispy bacon). Remove from the oven and, using tongs, place the bacon on a paper-towel-lined plate to cool.

Kid's job! Lay out a bamboo mat. Lay out one sheet of seaweed on the mat. Put one cup of rice on top of the seaweed. Using clean hands, evenly spread the rice out on the seaweed, leaving space at the top and the bottom of the seaweed.

continued

Kid's job! Lay a strip of cooked bacon in the middle of the nori, then sprinkle your kale on top. Time to roll. Lift the bamboo mat edge that's closest to you, and tightly tuck and roll your sushi. Use a dab of water on the top edge of the nori border to seal. Slice the roll into rounds using a sharp knife.

Serve with soy sauce for dipping.

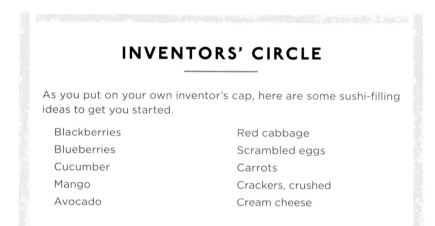

INVENTORS' CIRCLE

As you put on your own inventor's cap, here are some sushi-filling ideas to get you started.

Blackberries	Red cabbage
Blueberries	Scrambled eggs
Cucumber	Carrots
Mango	Crackers, crushed
Avocado	Cream cheese

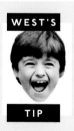

WEST'S TIP

Bacon and kale is one of my favorite combos. If you have any bacon, brown rice, and kale left over from making sushi, turn it into a stir-fry. Heat up a big stir-fry pan or wok over medium-high heat. Swirl some olive oil in it. Then throw in some crumbled cooked bacon, ripped-up raw kale, and cooked brown rice. Stir it for a few minutes. Taste. Pinch of salt? More bacon? More kale? I could eat a bucket of this.

CHICKEN À LA WEST

SERVES 4

2 boneless, skinless
chicken breasts
(about 12 ounces total)

2 tablespoons olive oil,
divided, plus more for
serving

1 tablespoon freshly
squeezed lime juice

1 tablespoon tamari

1 head butter lettuce,
trimmed, leaves
separated

Sea salt to taste

Chicken is one of those foods that takes on the flavor of whatever herbs, spices, or sauces you surround it with. West loves tamari, so a cubed chicken breast sautéed in some olive oil, lime juice, and tamari is a perfect protein for him. It can be eaten warm or cold, stuffed in a sandwich, wrapped in lettuce, served over rice, or just picked out of a bowl with little fingers.

Cube the chicken breasts and toss with 1 tablespoon olive oil, lime juice, tamari. Let stand 20 minutes at room temperature.

Place the lettuce leaves on a platter.

Heat the remaining olive oil in a medium pan over medium-high heat until hot but not smoking. Using a slotted spoon, transfer the chicken to the pan, sprinkle with salt, and cook for 3 to 5 minutes, stirring occasionally, until the chicken is just cooked through.

Transfer the chicken to a bowl. Fill each cup with chicken. Serve.

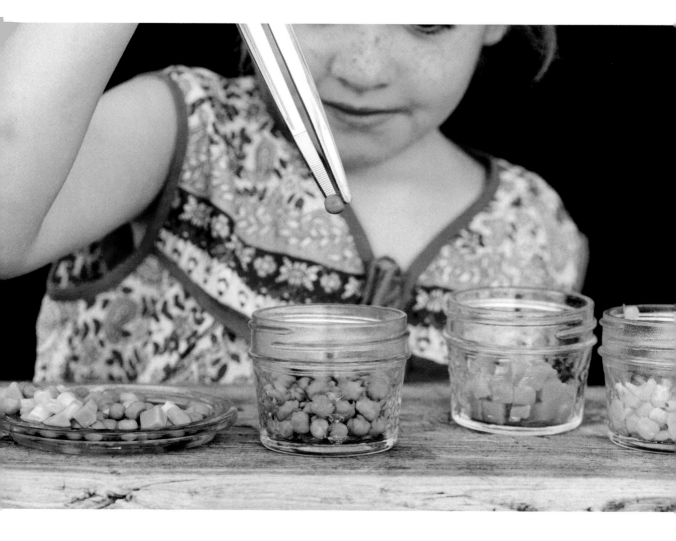

MAISON'S MASON JAR SHEPHERD'S PIE

SERVES 6

8 to 10 medium yellow potatoes or russet potatoes

Sea salt to taste

1 cup milk

6 tablespoons butter, divided

½ cup chopped onion

1 pound ground beef

2 cups frozen mixed veggies (carrots, peas, and corn)

1 cup grated Parmesan cheese

This is a twist on one of Misha's favorite childhood meals—shepherd's pie. This is a perfect opportunity for kids to play with (and sort) colorful veggies. Since playing with veggies tends to make kids more keen to eat them, we say bust out those tweezers and get your kids tweezing peas.

Preheat the oven to 375°F.

Peel and quarter the potatoes. Put them in a large pot and cover with cool water along with some salt. Bring to a boil and cook for 15 to 20 minutes, or until tender. Drain the potatoes, then return them to the pot. Add the milk and 4 tablespoons of butter as well as a few big pinches of salt. Mash with a potato masher until most of the lumps are gone. Put some muscle into it! Set aside.

Melt the remaining 2 tablespoons butter in a large sauté pan. Add the onion and salt. Sauté, stirring occasionally, for 5 minutes, or until the onions are tender and translucent. Add the beef, breaking it up with a spatula. Cook 7 to 9 minutes, until the beef has browned. Salt to taste.

Kid's job! Make your layers colorful: dump the frozen veggies out onto a clean counter and, using tweezers, divvy up the colors into piles—carrots, corn, and peas. Put a layer of beef in each of six 8-ounce mason jars, then add a layer of peas, a layer of carrots, a layer of corn, and top with mashed potatoes. Sprinkle cheese on top.

Put the jars onto a sheet pan and slide into the oven for 20 minutes, or until the cheese is melty and browned and the layers are warmed through. The jars will be hot—so let them cool for a few minutes before serving to kids.

STUFFED SWEET BABY BELLS

SERVES 4

16 baby bell peppers
(about 12 ounces total)

½ pound ground turkey

1 finely chopped scallion
(white and green parts)

½ teaspoon minced
ginger

1 garlic clove, smashed
and minced

1 teaspoon soy sauce

¼ teaspoon sea salt

DIPPING SAUCE

2 tablespoons
sesame oil

2 tablespoons rice
vinegar

1 tablespoon soy sauce

½ small clove garlic,
smashed and minced

¼ teaspoon minced
ginger

½ scallion (white part
only), finely chopped

Ever wonder what to make with those adorable mini peppers? Sure, they're cute, but what do you *do* with them? They're too small to slice, too seedy to just pop in your mouth. We decided to stuff them. They're perfect kid-size peppers. Another perfect little veggie pocket to fill.

Bring a few inches of water to a boil in a pot equipped with a steamer basket and a tight-fitting lid. Keep the basket out of the pot—you'll be snuggling your stuffed peppers into it before putting it over the boiling water.

Kid's job! Prep the peppers: cut the tops off the peppers. Scrape out the seeds with a small spoon or your fingers, then rinse the insides to remove any sneaky lingering seeds.

Make the filling: combine the ground turkey, scallion, ginger, garlic, soy sauce, and salt in a bowl and mix.

Fill the peppers: stuff a little bit of the turkey mixture into each tiny pepper. Snuggle the stuffed peppers into the steamer basket—it's okay if it's a snug fit. Place the steamer in the pot over the boiling water and cover. Steam 7 to 8 minutes, or until the turkey is cooked.

Kid's job! Meanwhile, to make the dipping sauce, combine all ingredients in a small bowl and whisk. Divide the sauce among four small dipping bowls. Dunk your peppers and enjoy.

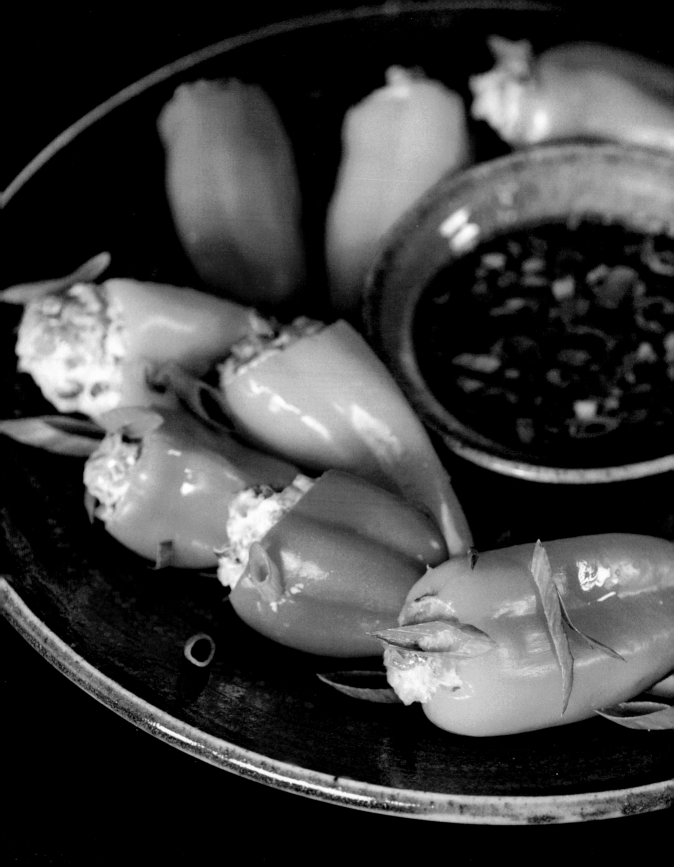

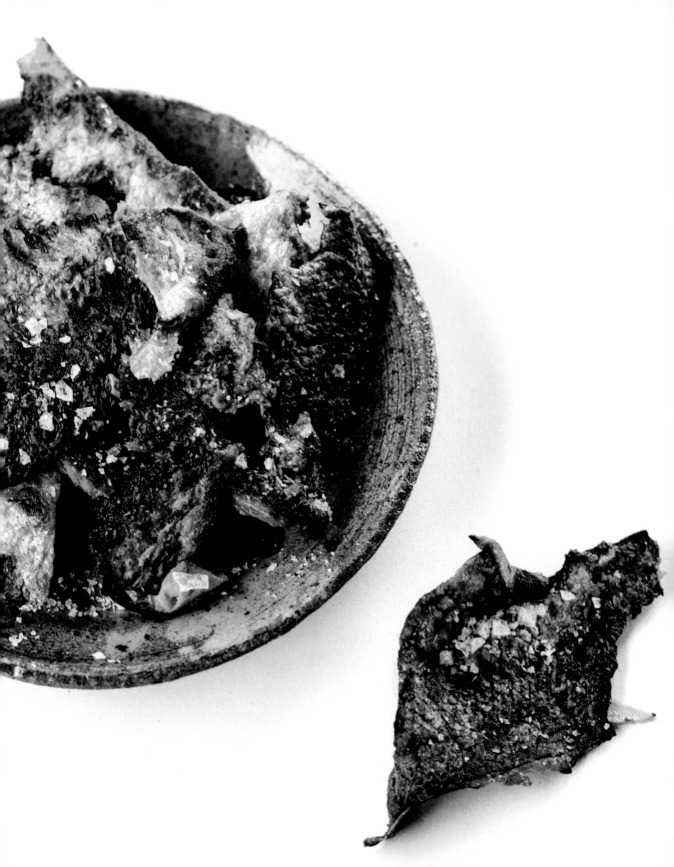

SALMON SKIN CHIPS

SERVES 2

1 salmon fillet, skin on,
pin bones removed
(about 12 ounces)

1 teaspoon sea salt

1 tablespoon vegetable
oil or ghee

West was a huge fan of salmon when he was two years old. Then suddenly, he shut down to salmon. But even at the height of his I-Hate-Salmon™ phase, he continued to adore the salty, crispy skin. If you're stuck with a fish-resister and you're making salmon for yourselves, try crisping the skin for the kids.

Preheat the oven to broil.

Kid's job! The trick here is a very dry fish. Pat your salmon dry thoroughly before cooking. Season the skin with a generous amount of salt and oil.

Put salmon on a greased cookie sheet skin side up. Place in the oven on broil for 3 minutes.

Remove from the oven. Turn the oven down to 350°F.

Let salmon cool for a minute, then peel the skin off. Place the skin (dry side down) on a new, lightly greased baking sheet and put it back into the oven.

Lay the salmon meat on a separate pan and pop back in the oven. Remove the skin chip from the oven after 8 minutes at 350°F. Let the salmon meat bake for 2 to 3 more minutes, until cooked through.

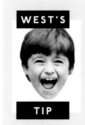

WEST'S TIP

Munch your salmon skin. Listen closely. Does it have a crunch louder than that of a potato chip? Did you know that salmon skin is packed with brain-building nutrients? Do you feel smarter after eating some? How does it taste on top of a potato chip?

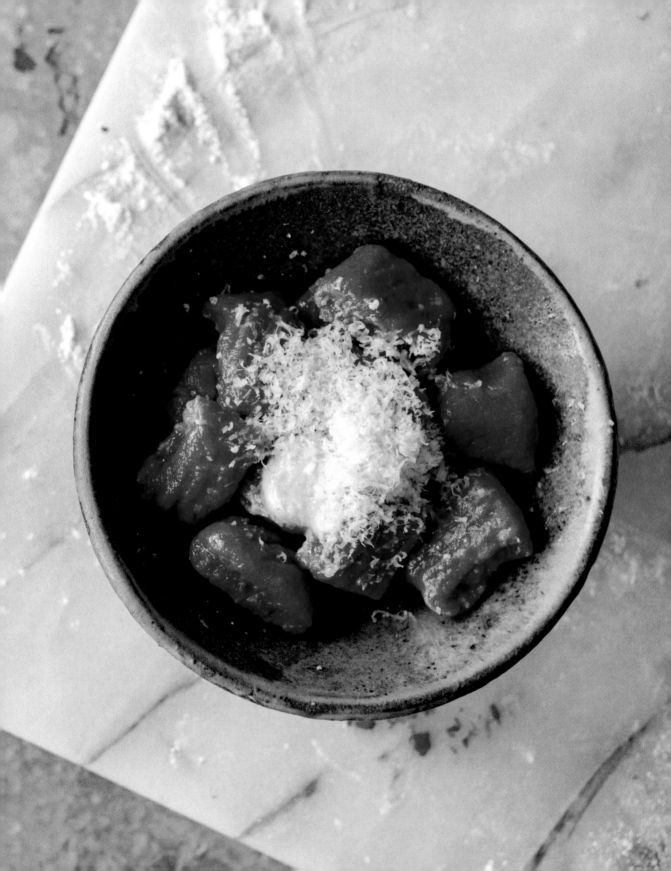

NOTHING BEETS PINK GNOCCHI!

SERVES 4

2 medium raw beets
(about 8 ounces total)

¼ teaspoon sea salt

I tablespoon olive oil

I½ cups all-purpose
flour, plus more for
dusting

¾ cup coarsely grated
Parmesan cheese

I teaspoon coarse salt

I egg

I cup ricotta cheese

Butter or olive oil
for garnish

¼ cup finely grated
Parmesan cheese
for garnish

We'd always heard that gnocchi was such a challenging dish to make that you have to be a real pro to try it. West and Maison got inspired after reading a children's book in which the family makes gnocchi from scratch. They insisted we give it a shot. As it turns out, we loved doing it so much that we invented our own pink version. It's messy and extremely fun.

Put the beets in a small saucepan, cover with cold water, add a pinch of table salt, and bring to a gentle boil. Boil until you can insert a fork in the beet, about 10 minutes. When you try lifting the beet from the water, it should slide right off the fork. Drain and let cool. Rub away the skin with your fingers. Cut each beet in quarters, then transfer to a blender. Add olive oil and a wee bit of water to help it get going. Blend until smooth.

Mound the flour on a clean surface (and since we're working with beets, make sure your surface is stain resistant). Create a well in the middle of your flour mountain, add the coarsely grated Parmesan and salt, and crack in your egg. Break the yolk with a fork and stir, incorporating the flour and cheese into your egg center a little at a time. After about half your flour is incorporated, fold in the beet puree and ricotta.

Now it's time to start working it all together with your hands. Sprinkle the work surface with extra flour to keep it from sticking, then mix the dough by kneading and folding it until it's smooth and the color is even. Then sprinkle more flour on your work surface, put the dough on top, and cover with a bowl. Let it nap for 30 minutes. No "knead" to overmix. (Dad joke.)

continued

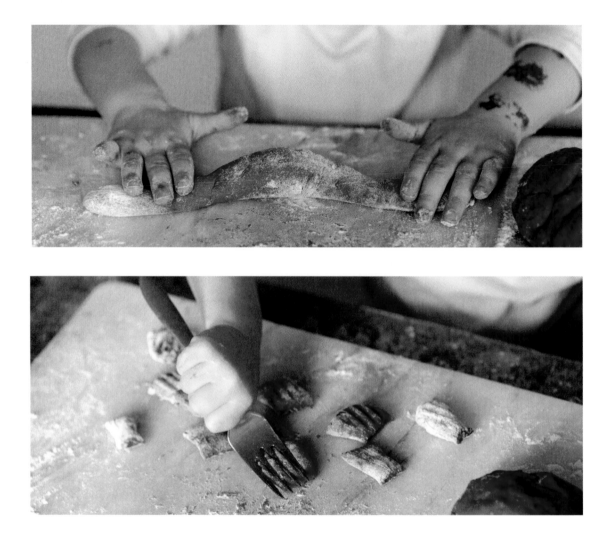

Kid's job! To make the gnocchi pieces, divide the dough into 4 sections and roll each section into ropes about the thickness of an adult's thumb. Using a kid knife, slice the ropes into ½-inch pieces. Press the tines of a fork gently into each piece to create some grooves and texture.

Bring a large pot of salted water to a boil. Gently add the gnocchi to the pot and stir.

Kid's job! When you see the gnocchi float, set the timer for 1 minute. When the timer beeps, use a slotted spoon to lift them out of the boiling water and transfer them to a bowl. Top with olive oil or butter, a sprinkle of salt, and Parmesan.

FAMILY CHALLENGE

TASTE TEST TIME!

In our family, we love taste tests. We do them because we think they're hilarious, but pediatric feeding experts recommend taste tests as a way to build confidence and trust while keeping a food experience positive and interactive.

If dinner includes a new food, invite your kids to conduct a taste test with it. We like to compare two versions of a new food. Perhaps chicken with and without soy sauce. Your kids' responses might tell you something about how they relate to food and offer some clues about how to segue into new dishes. Do they mostly describe the look, the colors, the textures, the sounds, or the flavors?

Words that are off-limits:

yucky

gross

disgusting

yummy

delicious

good

KIDS   Let's stick to words that describe the sensory experience of the food. How does the food feel in your mouth? What does this food remind you of? Does it feel crunchy in your mouth?

When you bite into the food, is it:

crunchy

smooth

soft

spicy

sweet

bitter

tangy

sour

crispy

chewy

salty

brightly colored

earthy smelling

nutty

loud when I bite it

doodley

green

?

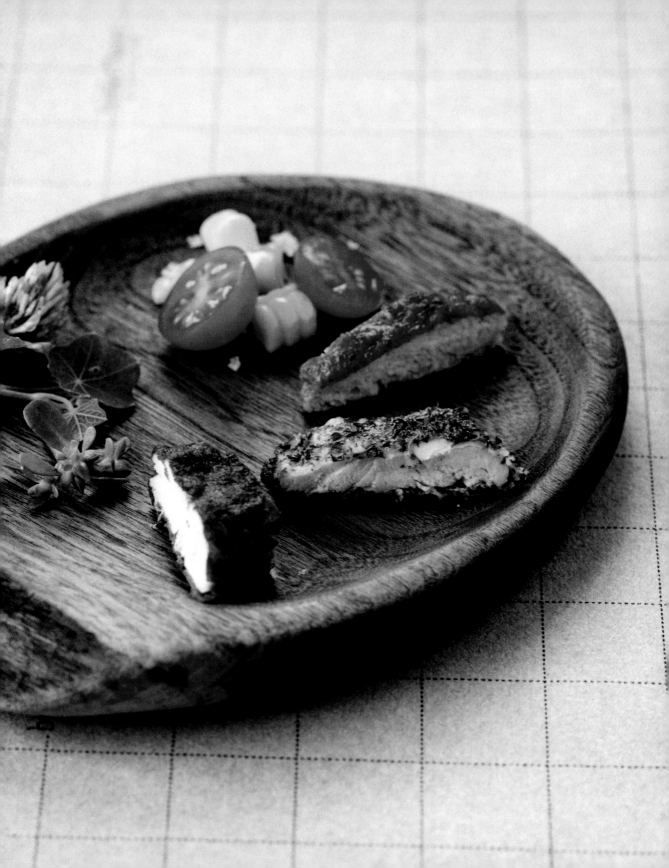

MIX 'N' MATCH "FRIED" CHICKEN

SERVES 4

2 eggs

¾ cup all-purpose flour, divided

2 tablespoons paprika

¾ teaspoon sea salt

2 tablespoons dried parsley

2 tablespoons cinnamon

4 boneless, skinless chicken breasts (about 20 ounces total)

½ stick (4 tablespoons) butter, melted

This chicken recipe offers a way for kids to experiment with three spices one at a time. It's also the kind of meal that they'll love making because it gives them an opportunity to dip and hammer. The end result is familiar to kids: it's a cousin of the infamous chicken tender, but these are covered in green and brown speckles, giving kids a chance to entertain the possibility that food with specks on it (i.e., herbs and spices) is not inherently terrifying.

Preheat the oven to 350°F. Grease a sheet pan and set it aside.

Set up a dredging station: grab four large shallow bowls or pie pans. Crack the eggs into one bowl, then break the yolks with a whisk or fork; gently whisk for a few seconds. This is your wet pan. Add ¼ cup of flour to each of the three other pie pans—these are your dry pans. Add the paprika and salt to one, the parsley and salt to another, and the cinnamon and salt to the third. Stir the flour mixtures so the seasonings are evenly distributed in each pan.

Cut each chicken breast into four strips. Put the strips between two sheets of plastic wrap, grab your mallet, and smash that meat till it's ¾ of an inch thick. Now you're ready to dredge and dip.

Kid's job! Dip those tenders: Lift one piece of chicken and dunk it into dry pan #1 to coat the meat on all sides, being sure to knock off any excess by giving it a shake, shake, shake. Now dunk it into the wet pan—the egg has something to hold on to since you coated the chicken in a little flour mix first! The final step: back into the dry pan #1. Give the chicken a good final coating, then gently knock off any excess. Lay your dredged chicken onto your greased sheet pan. Repeat with dry pan #2, and then dry pan #3.

Drizzle melted butter over each dredged piece of chicken before popping the pan into the oven. Bake for 25 to 35 minutes.

Adventure Recipe
MAKE-A-HUGE-MESS SANDWICH

SERVES 4

4 cups cooked spaghetti
with tomato sauce

8 slices
sandwich bread

Although the never-ending tornado that children bring to the kitchen can be trying for any parent, kids'-food experts say getting messy is an important way young kids get familiar with new foods. As annoying as the wreckage can be to clean up (Jelly on the dog? Egg yolk on the upholstery?), these savory and sweet catastrophes often lead to a willingness to try new foods. Pediatric expert Melanie Potock says, "Embrace the mess that naturally coincides with self-feeding, because at that very messy moment, your child is actively learning about food!" Taking her words to heart, and keeping a garden hose at the ready, we designed this sandwich to embrace that sentiment.

Kid's job! Put your saucy spaghetti between two bread slices.

Put on a white T-shirt. Eat your saucy spaghetti sandwich over a tarp or in the bathtub. Have a giggly mess of a good time.

The goal, of course, is to be completely covered in food.

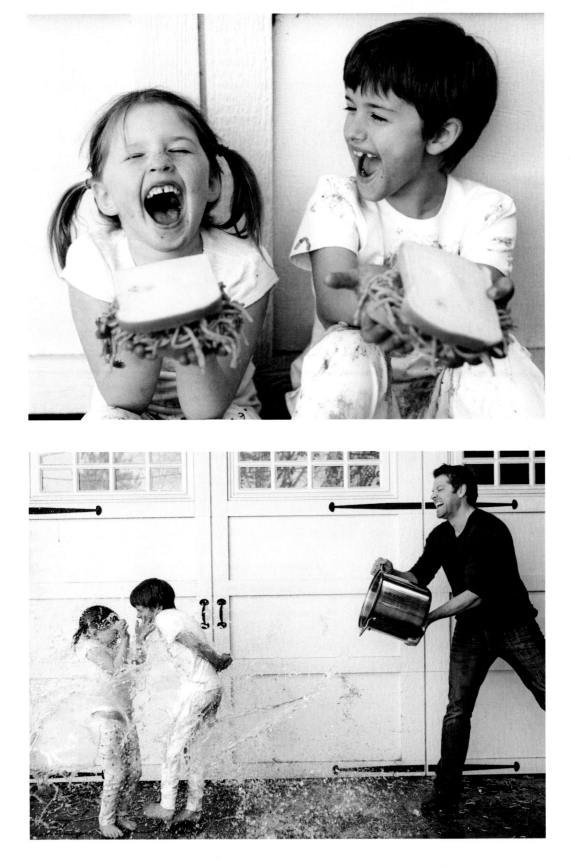

Pasta with Jam Sauce

RECIPES ONLY A KID COULD DREAM UP

West's signature dish, Pasta with Jam Sauce, is a nontraditional Thanksgiving dinner West invented when he was a toddler during a webisode of *Cooking Fast & Fresh with West*. Let your toddler go rogue in the kitchen: you'll likely witness culinary fearlessness.

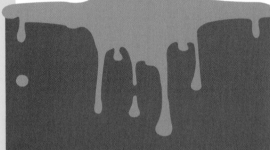

10 strawberry jam

"So many" tomato sauce from a can

5 inches carrot juice

All the orange juice in the refrigerator

1 bag chocolate chips

¾ bag Goldfish

8 inches fresh blackberries

1 whole Red Delicious apple, including stem and core, less three small bites

1 box wheel-shaped pasta

1 jar tomato sauce

Handful of popped popcorn

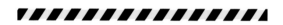

Mix all ingredients in a large bowl. Wearing goggles, beat vigorously with an electric hand mixer, one beater inside the bowl and the other outside it. Pour into a large pot and bring to a boil. Stir as desired. Boil until thick and brown.

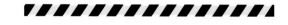

THE CRITICS CHIME IN

We challenged bona fide food critics around the world to taste and review West's Pasta with Jam Sauce. Several rose to the occasion. *San Francisco Chronicle* food critic Jonathan Kauffman generously called the dish "edible," noting that it "did not taste as much like vomit" as he expected. He admitted it was "too tangy," however, and "not really something anyone should eat, ever." Here's what other critics said about West's signature dish . . .

"I don't hate it."

> —Rick Nelson, restaurant critic
> for *Star Tribune* (Minneapolis)

"Collins's sauce is a dirty bomb aimed at America's Thanksgiving tables."

> —Matthew Amster-Burton, former
> food writer for *The Seattle Times*

"A potential parody (and lesson!) of foods that should never, ever, ever, ever get back together. If at all."

> —Chadwick Boyd, food and lifestyle
> expert for NBC, ABC, CBS,
> and the Food Network

"There's only one reasonable pairing with this unfortunate dish: Listerine. . . . Translation: this really sucks. It doesn't suck bad enough that I now hate all five-year-olds. But it sucks enough to say that five-year-olds should not be given carte blanche when it comes to designing recipes. Did I hate this dish? *Hate* is a strong word. But it's not strong enough. I despised this dish. I hope it doesn't haunt me until the day I die, though I fear it will."

> —Blair Robertson, former restaurant
> critic for *The Sacramento Bee*

"I don't think I would want to eat a whole bowl of this, but that's my adult palate talking."

> —Robin Garr, former food and travel
> writer for the *New York Times*

"Sad to see so many wonderful ingredients used in such an inedible way."

> —Betsy Cohen, blogger of
> *Desserts Required*

"A bland, unpalatable mélange of crunchy, undercooked pasta, chocolate, and berry jam . . ."

> —Wynter Holden, food critic for
> *Phoenix* magazine

"West creates industry waves via his ad-hoc cooking style, which sees him throwing in a nibbled whole apple, some leftover Goldfish crackers, and even some choc chips for good measure. Although West certainly wouldn't win the award for tidiest chef, Jamie Oliver didn't become a food icon via mixing safely with a spoon; it's all about getting amongst it and getting the feeling of the food from the get-go. West's Pasta with Jam Sauce is as original as it could get, and although it may not become an acclaimed gourmand Michelin-star coveted meal, it could easily become a kid-friendly staple . . ."

> —Emma McNamara, former
> food reviewer for *The Urban List*
> (Sydney, Australia)

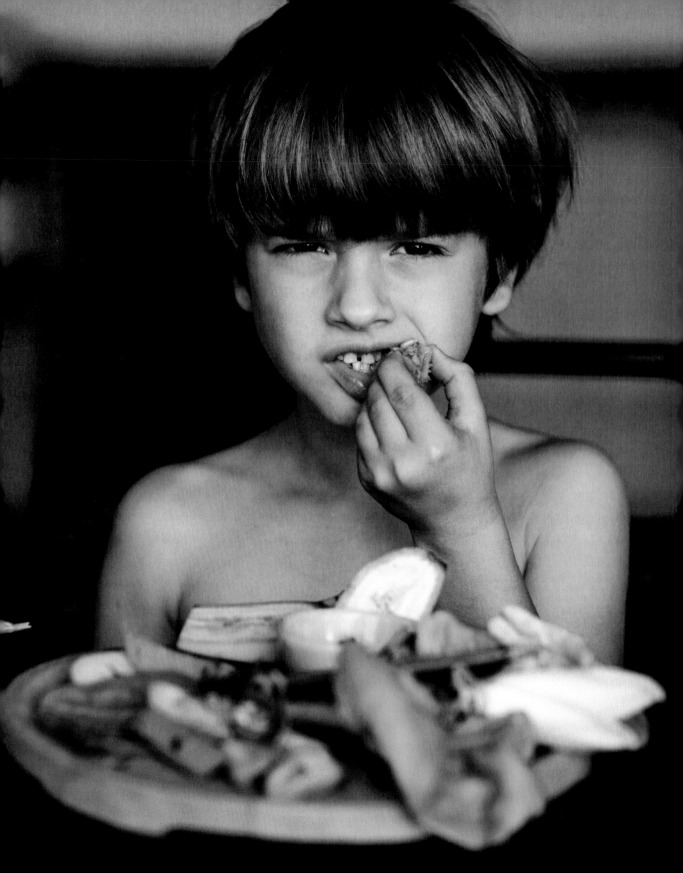

REINVENTING
THE SNACK...
SALAD POPSICLES,
ANYONE?

When our son was a toddler, if he went for a few hours without eating, he'd spiral into a grouchy fit. In self-defense, we developed a habit of stuffing crackers into his mouth from the moment he woke up in the morning till we tucked him in at night. Unsurprisingly, he stopped eating at mealtimes and lost interest in trying new foods.

Our family's all-day grazing isn't unique. Grazing has become the cornerstone American eating pattern, especially for children. We're raising a generation of snackers. Many American kids snack three to six times a day, and some eat almost constantly all day long.

A study of more than thirty-one thousand kids found that the average US kid consumes roughly six hundred calories per day from snacks—nearly one-third of their daily calories. If kids were consuming a wide variety of whole food snacks, that'd be one thing. But American kids are snacking primarily on desserts like cookies and cakes (the number one source of snack food) and on salty processed foods like chips and pretzels (the second most popular snack category).

One of the downsides of these common snacks is that they're low in fiber and protein, and high in sugar. Did you know that a single serving of Yoplait yogurt contains as much sugar as a Snickers bar? Snacks for children have turned into a multibillion-dollar industry that shamelessly markets neon-colored artificial foods to kids and preys on their affinity for superheroes. In the late 1990s, the food giant General Mills tested the market for a sugar-loaded "yogurt" that could be squeezed directly into mouths without the inconvenience of a spoon—it was the first yogurt designed specifically for kids. The company made $100 million in year one from that culinary masterpiece, and has marketed Go-Gurt as a family pantry necessity ever since. This kind of flavor-engineered, ready-made snack in a brightly colored package is ubiquitous in American culture.

For parents, it's easy to cling to these quick snacks as if your life depends on them. They're just so convenient.

You know what else is a convenient grab-and-go snack? An apple. Or a carrot. Or a handful of almonds. There are plenty of homemade snacks that are inexpensive and quick, and that kids can learn to love.

For the most part, we think of snacks as mini meals rather than treats, and we use fresh fruits and vegetables when we can. We set up simple snack plates with several options—and children can choose what to eat from what we've offered. Kids don't get to demand any particular snack. Sure, if they've got a vision for inventing a new snack from the ingredients we stock at home, we're game, but usually *we* serve the snacks.

This chapter offers fun, wholesome snack ideas and inspiration—including some that are just as portable and easy as Goldfish. We've divided our recipes into two sections:

- **HOME SNACKS:** Translation—messy. Best eaten sitting at a table.

- **GRAB AND GOS:** For grabbing and going.

We've focused on snacks that taste great and are fun to make (and eat) with kids and that provide their little bodies with steady streams of energy; no crashes, no bouncing off the walls, no tantrums. Let the snacking begin.

Home Snacks

NIBBLES

We don't advise eating these upside down. Or in a stroller. You may even want to spread out a tarp (or bib) for these bad boys, because they can get messy.

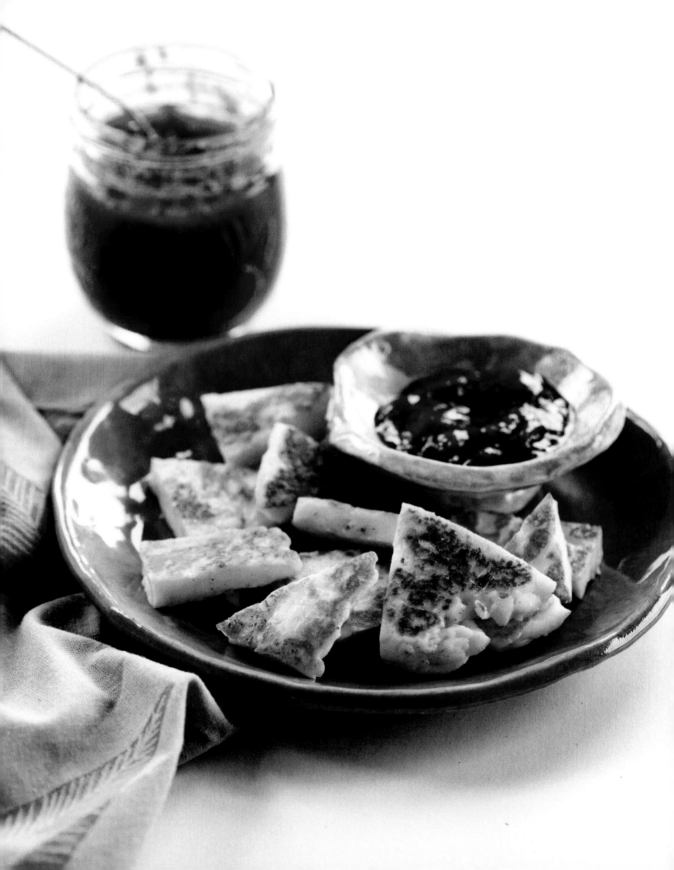

SQUEAKY CHEESE
WITH JAM SAUCE

SERVES 4

½ cup chopped fresh strawberries

½ cup chopped fresh rhubarb

¼ cup maple syrup

¼ cup water

2 tablespoons olive oil

7 ounces presliced halloumi cheese

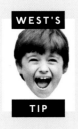

WEST'S TIP

When you bite into this cheese, listen carefully . . . can you hear it squeak between your teeth? It sounds like sneakers on a basketball court!

Many American parents believe their kids will only eat bland, orange-colored cheese. Maybe your kid isn't ready to gnaw a hunk of Roquefort or stinky blue (ours aren't there yet), but this recipe offers an approachable foray into the territory of new types of cheese. Instead of defaulting to orange cheese for kids, we decided not to stock it at home and instead keep an assortment of cheeses. All cheese-tasting expeditions should begin with a wondrous salty cheese called halloumi, which is a blend of sheep's, goat's, and cow's milk. It's originally from Cyprus, but even Trader Joe's carries it now. Halloumi has a unique texture and can be grilled, sautéed, or fried without melting. Bonus: the whole family can enjoy the squeaky sounds this cheese makes when bitten.

To make the jam, combine the berries, rhubarb, maple syrup, and water in a medium pot over medium heat. Bring to a boil, then reduce the heat to low and simmer for about 40 minutes. Stir occasionally. Cover and remove from heat while you prepare the cheese.

Heat the olive oil in a large skillet over medium-high heat until hot but not smoking. Arrange the cheese slices in the skillet in a single layer. Wait 30 seconds or so before checking the undersides for golden-brown. It may take a few minutes . . . then flip. Cook the other side until golden brown. Let the slices cool a bit before biting into this yummy salty cheese. Dip liberally in warm jam sauce.

HOT APPLES

SERVES 4 TO 6

4 apples (Fuji and Gala are our favorites for this)

¼ teaspoon cinnamon

I vanilla bean

Our family is passionate about apple season. We pick apples by the bushel: then we dehydrate them to make apple chips, bake them, and slice and dip them in assorted nut butters. We love this easy recipe, and it fills our entire house with a homey, delicious aroma as it bubbles and bakes. This naturally sweet treat is so simple that the most difficult thing will be waiting for it to cool down enough to eat.

Preheat the oven to 350°F.

Kid's job! Using a swivel peeler and a kid-safe knife, peel, core, and cut your apples into 2-inch chunks. Pile the chunks into a medium casserole dish and sprinkle with the cinnamon. Cut the vanilla bean in half lengthwise. Reserve one half for another use. Scrape the insides of the other half into the casserole, then add the empty bean carcass. Mix thoroughly.

Cover the casserole with foil and bake for 1 hour. Remove the casserole from the oven and uncover. Let the apples cool for at least 5 minutes.

Once cool enough to eat, the apples will be spoon-tender. Dig in.

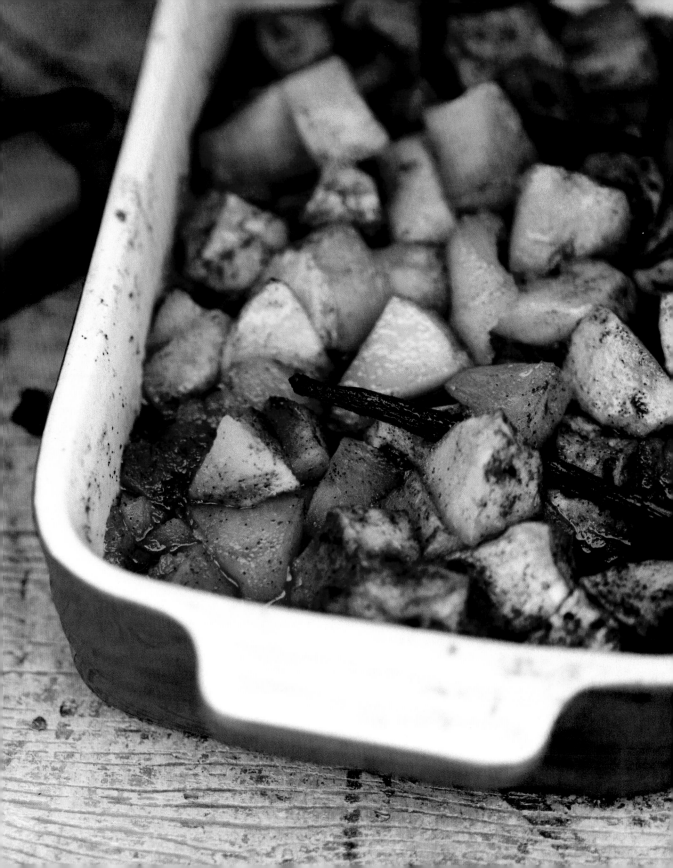

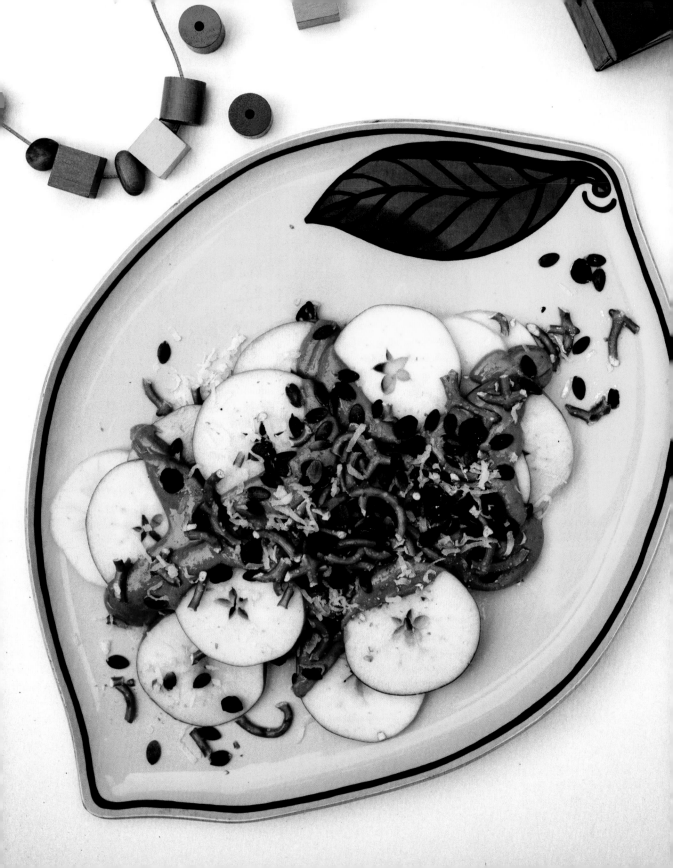

APPLE NACHOS

SERVES 2 TO 4

2 to 3 apples

½ lemon

2 tablespoons peanut butter (the old-fashioned sugar-free kind you have to stir)

Small handful of raisins

Small handful of raw pumpkin seeds

Small handful of flaked unsweetened coconut

Small handful of pretzels, crushed

This sweet version of the halftime classic gives your little ones all the fun of nachos with a nutty protein boost.

Lay each apple on its side and slice it into rounds right through the core. You should have about 8 slices per apple. Make your slices thin like chips but thick enough to hold the toppings. Squeeze the lemon over the slices so they don't brown. Pluck out the seeds, revealing the pretty star/flower-shaped center of each apple slice.

Kid's job! Stir 1 tablespoon of water into your peanut butter until it's thin enough to drizzle. Pile your apple "chips" on a plate. Drizzle the peanut butter over the top. Sprinkle on raisins, pumpkin seeds, coconut flakes, and crushed pretzels.

FIND THE APPLE OF YOUR EYE

There are more than 2,500 varieties of apples in the world. Take a tour of your local farmers' market during apple season and taste one of each available variety. Some are crisp; some are sweet; others are tart. Do a blind tasting to figure out which one is your favorite. If you could rename your favorite apple, what would you call it?

SPOON BREAD

SERVES 6 TO 8

1½ cups finely ground cornmeal

2 teaspoons baking powder

Few pinches of sea salt

I cup milk

I tablespoon honey, plus more for drizzling

2 eggs, separated

4 tablespoons butter, plus more for serving

West swears this bread tastes like buttered popcorn. He's right. We spoon it out warm from a cast-iron pan straight into our mouths.

Preheat the oven to 375°F.

Whisk together the cornmeal, baking powder, and salt in a large bowl.

In a medium saucepan over low heat, gently warm the milk. Remove from heat and stir in the honey until it dissolves. Whisk in the egg yolks, then fold the mixture into the cornmeal mixture until just combined.

Melt the butter in a 9-inch cast-iron skillet. Brush it around the bottom and sides of a medium skillet so the entire surface is coated. Pour the excess into the batter and stir.

Beat the egg whites until fluffy. Using a spatula, gently fold the egg whites into the cornmeal batter. You want to keep the batter fluffy and the egg whites inflated so they help the bread rise a bit.

Spread the batter evenly inside the buttered skillet. Bake for 20 minutes, or until golden. Remove the pan from the oven and top the bread with butter and drizzles of honey while it's still hot. Serve warm.

WHIP LIKE WEST

While traditional recipes call for egg whites to be beaten with an electric mixer, West likes pouring them into a plastic bottle with a tight-fitting cap. The bottle needs to be totally dry inside. Now play catch with the bottle. Shake it wildly. Keep going until the eggs turn foamy and stiff.

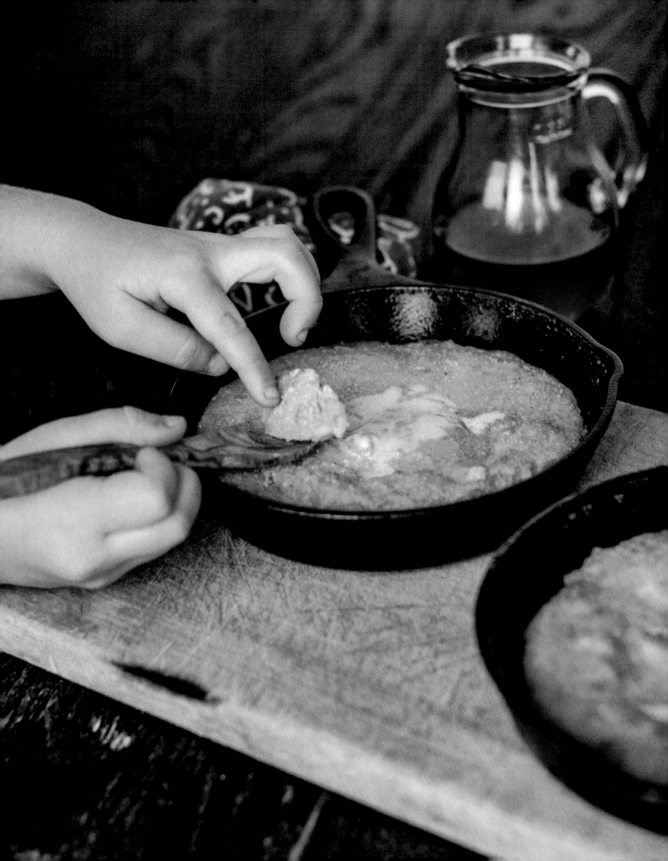

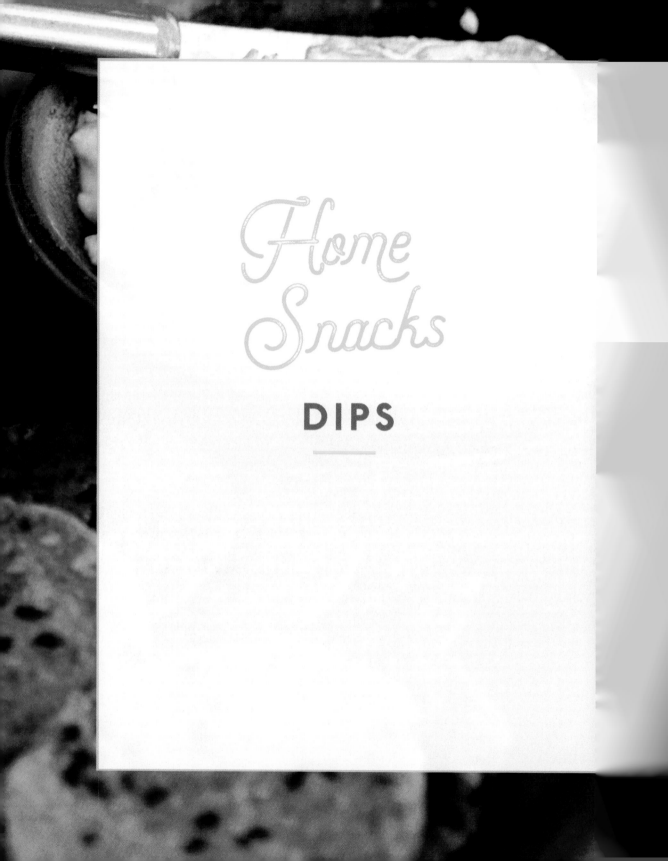

Home Snacks

DIPS

PINK HUMMUS

SERVES 4 TO 6

1 small raw beet

1 clove garlic, smashed and peeled

1 15-ounce can chickpeas, drained and rinsed

Zest and juice of 1 lemon

1 tablespoon tahini

Sea salt to taste

¼ cup olive oil

Homemade hummus is quick and fun to make. A few rounds in the food processor, and you're good to go. This version is like ordinary hummus, only naturally pink, from beets.

Peel the raw beet. Roughly chop the beet and place it in a food processor.

Add the garlic, chickpeas, lemon zest and juice, tahini, and salt. Whirr until well blended. Then on low speed, stream in the olive oil while the processor is running. Stop and scrape down the sides of the bowl and taste.

ZIP-LOCK GUAC

SERVES 3 TO 4

1 ripe avocado

Juice of 1 lime or lemon

Pinch of sea salt

Every parent knows that children cherish any opportunity to squeeze and squish and mash. So give them an avocado to squish in a sealed plastic bag. All that squeezing fun might intrigue them so much that they'll be game to taste this simple guacamole.

Grown-ups: cut the avocado open. Scoop it out of the peel and throw the flesh into a strong zip-lock bag. Add the juice, and salt. Squeeze the air from your bag and zip it up.

Kid's job! Mash your 'mole. Mash, mash, mash by hand until very smooth.

Snip off one of the bottom corners of the bag and squeeze your zip-lock guacamole into a bowl, like it's frosting.

Serve with crackers or on toast.

Adventure Recipe
YOGURT CHEESE DIP

SERVES 4

32 ounces full-fat plain yogurt

Sea salt to taste

1 sprig fresh dill

Cheese has always seemed too intimidating to make at home. Then we found this magical way of turning yogurt into cheese. Start with a tub of plain yogurt and end up with a thick spread or dip that you can customize to be as sweet or savory. Kids can do every step of this process. The only special equipment you'll need is a piece of cheesecloth for straining.

Fit a strainer over a large bowl, leaving a couple of inches between the bottom of the strainer and the bottom of the bowl. Fold an 18 × 36-inch piece of cheesecloth into a large square and drape it over the strainer. You should have 2 layers of cheesecloth with some length hanging over the strainer on each side. Dump the yogurt into the cheesecloth and fold over the excess to cover. Set the bowl in the refrigerator and leave it overnight. By morning you'll see the whey has separated from the yogurt, leaving a thick and spreadable yogurt cheese. West loves to drink the whey.

Add your mix-ins. Taste the plain cheese, add salt. Use scissors to snip the fresh dill into tiny green flecks. Sprinkle a few green flecks into the yogurt cheese.

Serve on toast, over crackers, in wraps, in bowls, or on top of pancakes.

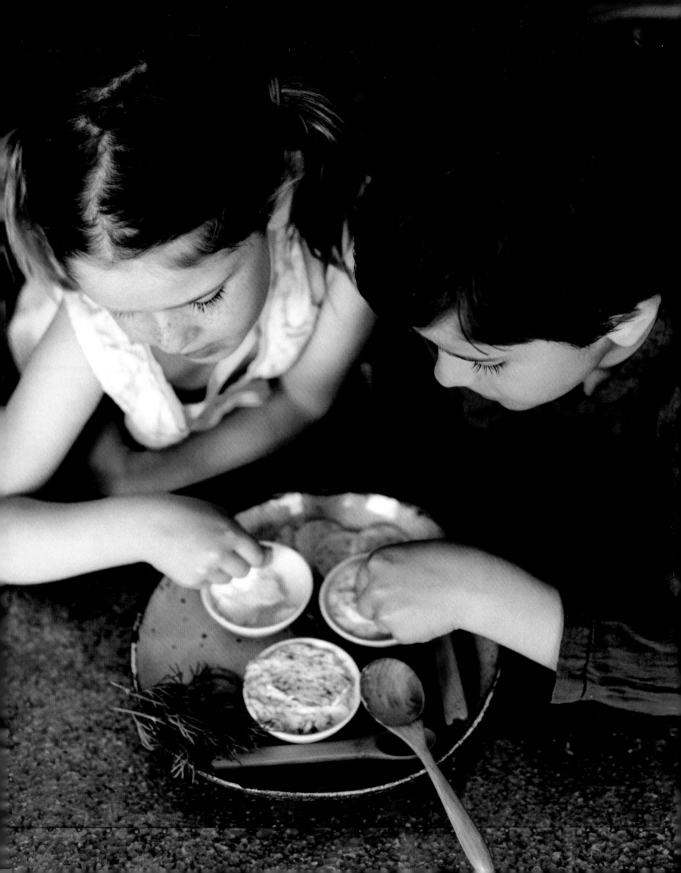

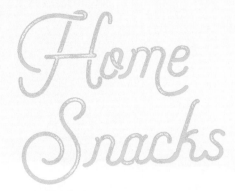

Home Snacks

TOASTS

There's something especially comforting about the smell of toast. In our family, we like to use whole-grain bread packed with little seeds (check the package—most breads sold at grocery stores these days contain sugar, cane syrup, and over-processed flours). The anticarb frenzy has turned plenty of adults against toast, but 100% real whole-grain toast is a hearty and healthful treat. Plus, toast makes a perfect platform for new flavors and texture combinations.

BABT
(BACON, AVOCADO, AND BLUEBERRY TOAST)

SERVES 1

2 strips bacon

1 slice bread

¼ pitted ripe avocado

Handful of blueberries

Lemon wedge

Sea salt to taste

Preheat the oven to 375°F.

Lay the bacon strips in a single layer on a cookie sheet. Bake for 15 minutes, or a little longer if you like extra-crisp bacon. Using tongs, lift the strips out of the rendered bacon fat and let them cool on paper towels.

Kid's job! Toast your bread slice. Scoop out your avocado right on top, using a fork to mash the avo all the way to the edges for a nice even layer. Make an X out of the bacon strips and dot with blueberries. The berries may roll around a little, so push them right into the avocado to help them stay put. Squeeze the lemon wedge over the creation and sprinkle with salt.

GRASSY FIELD TOAST

SERVES 1

1 unpeeled fresh ripe pear

3 leaves baby spinach

1 slice bread

1 to 2 teaspoons almond butter

Slice off a chunk from the pear, then cut it into small dice. You should have ¼ cup. Set aside.

Stack the spinach leaves one on top of the other, roll them tightly to form a "cigar," then slice them horizontally into thin ribbons, or "blades of grass." Set aside.

Kid's job! Toast the bread, then spread it with the almond butter. Sprinkle the field of spinach on top of the almond butter, then sprinkle the pear pieces on top.

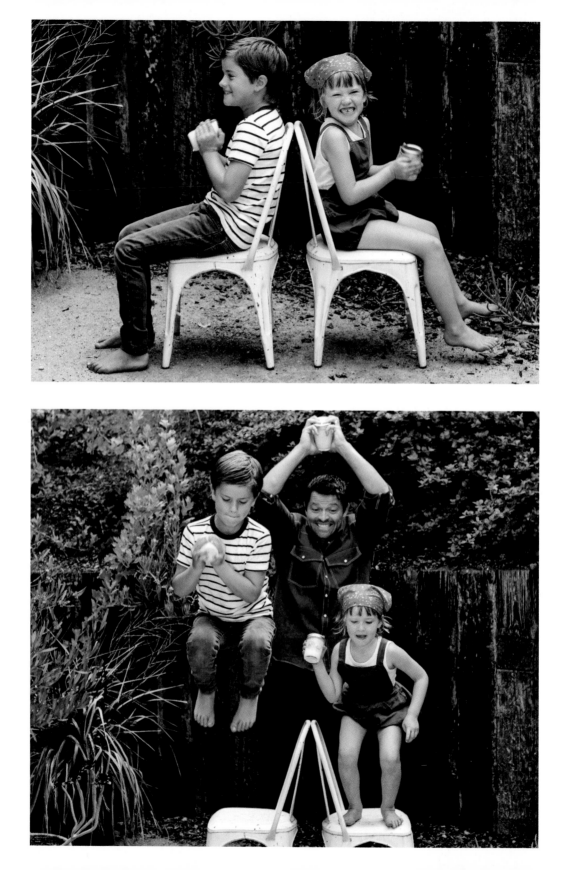

HOP AND SHAKE BUTTER

SERVES 6

1 pint heavy whipping cream

Sea salt to taste

If you want toast without all the bells and whistles, how about simply topping it with homemade butter? We love making our own butter. Not only is it more delicious than store-bought, it's also easy. Plus, kids (and, let's face it, adults) find it satisfying to transform a liquid into a solid by jumping, hopping, and shaking. You'll need a small jar with a snug-fitting lid, such as a pint-size pickle jar, a baby food jar, or a four-ounce mason jar. The more heavy cream you use, the longer it takes, so for very young kids, we start with small baby food jars.

Kid's job! First things first: fill your jar halfway with cream. Screw the lid on tightly.

Shake it up. Now shake it, shake it, baby. It's going to take some endurance. The cream will turn into whipped cream, first with soft peaks, then with stiff peaks. You may need to do a taste test. Did we say you were done after you tasted? Nope. Keep going. Shake it, baby. Now shake it while jumping on one foot. Now shake it while singing your favorite song. Tired of shaking? Too bad—keep shaking. The more you hop and shake, the better the butter.

When you start to hear sloshing and you feel solid stuff slamming on the sides of the jar, you're nearly there. Once you see clear liquid separating from the butter, you're done. Pour off the clear liquid (it's buttermilk) and give it a taste.

After you've poured out the buttermilk, use a rubber spatula to scrape out the butter. Then grab it with your hands and shape it into a ball under cold running water until the water runs clear. Shake off extra water from your butter ball and place it in a bowl. Now salt your butter. Spread your butter into ramekins and serve. Plain homemade butter will stay fresh in a crock on your countertop for five to seven days and in the fridge for seven to ten days.

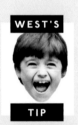

WEST'S

TIP

I like to add honey and a handful of fresh strawberries to my homemade butter. We mix these ingredients into the butter with a spoon. Or you can swirl in your favorite jam to make marbled butter.

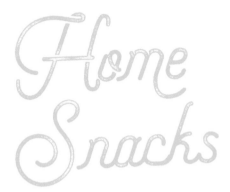

Home Snacks

MAISON'S
SALAD POPSICLES

When we asked Maison what flavor popsicle she wanted to make, she didn't hesitate: salad. We know what you're thinking, but they're really good. Store-bought pops are usually a mixture of juice, sugar, and preservatives. Our homemade pops incorporate chunks of fruits and veggies (including the fiber that's been stripped out of most prepackaged pops) for a uniquely green twist on a classic.

Each recipe makes six 3-ounce pops.

For each recipe, combine all ingredients in a blender or food processor and blend until smooth. Pour the puree into popsicle molds with built-in sticks. Freeze for 5 hours, then enjoy.

CARROT-ORANGE CREAMSICLE

½ peeled banana

½ peeled carrot

1 peeled orange
(pluck out the seeds)

1½ cups orange juice

½ cup plain yogurt

1 teaspoon vanilla
extract

GREEN SALAD POP

½ cup unpeeled
cucumber chunks

½ cup tightly packed
baby spinach leaves

½ cup green
honeydew melon
chunks

1½ cups apple juice

¼ cup plain yogurt

PINEAPPLE SALAD POP

½ cup peeled
kiwifruit chunks

1 cup tightly packed
baby spinach leaves

½ cup canned, fresh,
or frozen pineapple
chunks

1½ cups apple juice

SALTY PEANUT POP

½ peeled banana

½ cup peanut
butter (smooth
old-fashioned kind
without sugar or
palm oil)

2 tablespoons
soy sauce

¼ cup honey

1½ cups coconut milk

Pinch of sea salt

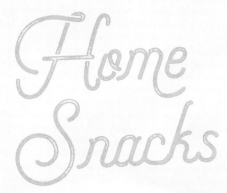

Home Snacks

SMOOTHIES

Smoothies offer so many opportunities for you to get creative. On the following pages you'll find some of our family's favorite protein-rich blends.

Each recipe serves four.

For each recipe, combine all the ingredients in a blender and zap until smooth.

CHOOSE-YOUR-OWN-ADVENTURE SMOOTHIE

SERVES 4

Start with these ingredients:

1 frozen banana

3 tablespoons unsalted nut butter

4 pitted dates

½ cup frozen or fresh spinach

¾ cup milk or nut milk

Smoothies can be overly sweet and syrupy. Or they can be hearty snacks packed with protein, fresh produce, and fiber. Start with our family's protein-rich smoothie base. Lay out some optional add-ins and encourage your kids to go wild. They'll need adult supervision to operate the blender. It helps to have a workhorse blender that can handle everything from nuts to raw roots. (West once threw raw butternut squash into the blender.)

Kid's job! Choose optional add-ins:

Chia seeds

Unsalted pecans, almonds, walnuts, peanuts, or pumpkin seeds

Frozen blueberries, mangoes, or strawberries

Cinnamon

Salad greens

Vanilla

Yogurt

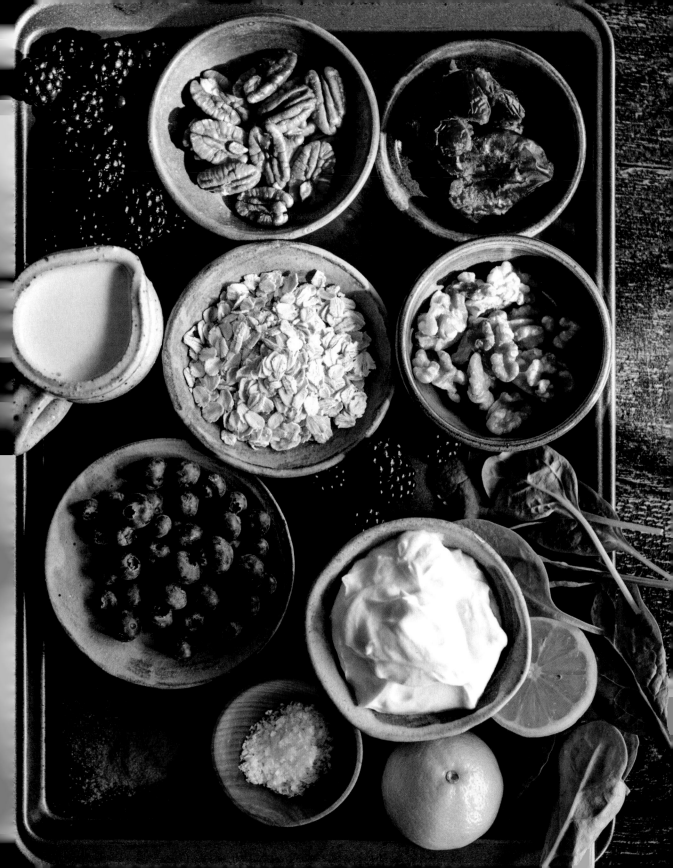

MISHA'S BLACKBERRY PIE SMOOTHIE

3 dried pitted dates, roughly chopped

¼ cup fresh blackberries

¼ cup fresh blueberries

¼ cup rolled oats

¼ cup walnut halves

¼ cup pecan halves

⅓ cup spinach leaves

½ teaspoon cinnamon

Juice of ½ lemon

½ cup plain yogurt

½ cup milk

½ cup ice cubes

WEST'S MINTY CHOCOLATE SMOOTHIE

3 dried pitted dates, roughly chopped

I cup firmly packed torn destemmed kale leaves

I cup firmly packed baby spinach leaves

¼ cup firmly packed fresh mint leaves

¼ cup cashews

I tablespoon unsweetened cocoa powder

I teaspoon vanilla extract

½ cup plain yogurt

½ cup milk

½ cup ice cubes

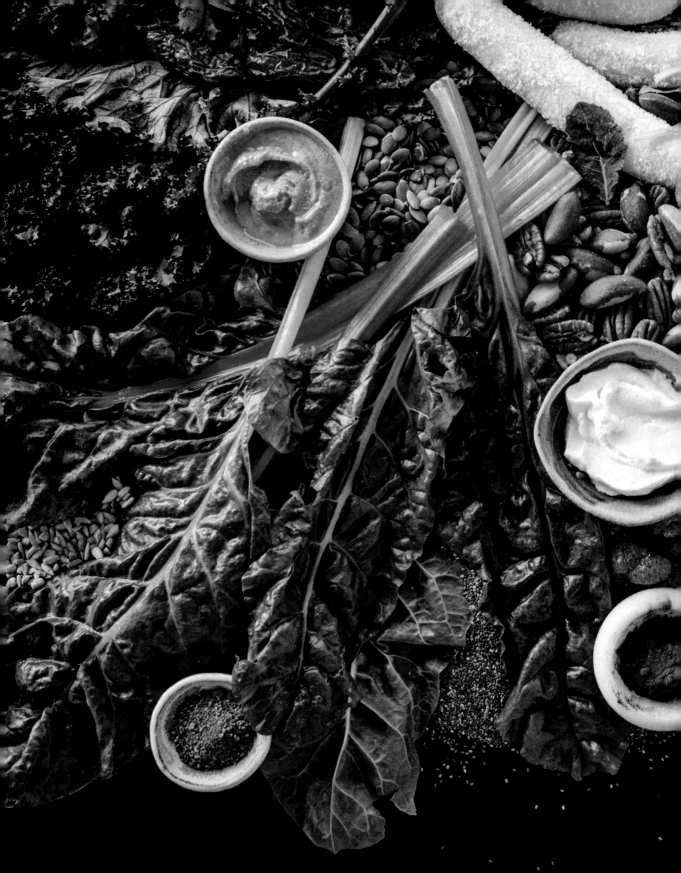

THE SECRETS OF OUR SMOOTHIE PANTRY

Here are some of the ingredients we keep on hand for smoothie madness. With this smoothie pantry, you can invent some seriously delicious concoctions . . .

- *Frozen baby spinach leaves (buy fresh prewashed leaves, then freeze 'em)*

- *Fresh destemmed kale leaves (buy them fresh, then freeze 'em)*

- *Chia seeds*

- *Raw sunflower seeds*

- *Raw pumpkin seeds*

- *Unsalted raw pecans, walnuts, almonds, cashews, and peanuts*

- *Frozen bananas (peel 'em, then freeze 'em)*

- *Old-fashioned sugar-free peanut butter that you have to stir*

- *Unsweetened cocoa powder*

- *Frozen berries of all kinds (blueberries, strawberries)*

- *Plain yogurt*

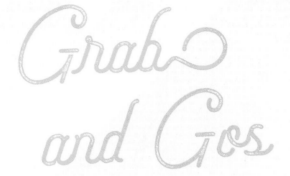

Grab and Gos

These compact snacks take some prep, but they're easy to grab as you're walking out the door.

BANANA OATMEAL PUCKS

MAKES 16 TO 18

2 small very ripe bananas

1 cup rolled oats

1 teaspoon vanilla extract

½ cup chopped walnuts

½ cup raisins

Two out of two of our children have found this combination of creamy-licious bananas mixed with raisins, nuts, and oats to be 100 percent irre-sistible. Not only are they a mushy delight for kids to help make, they also only take a few minutes in the oven until they're ready to go.

Preheat the oven to 350°F. Grease a cookie sheet and set aside.

Kid's job! Mash it up. In a medium mixing bowl, using a potato masher or fork, mash the bananas thoroughly. Stir in the oats, vanilla, nuts, and raisins.

Kid's job! Roll the mixture into rounds the size of Ping-Pong balls and place them on the greased cookie sheet. Smash them down with your hand to make them a bit flat. Bake for 10 minutes. Remove from the oven. Let cool and store in an airtight container.

THE MOUNTAINEER'S SNACK

MAKES 8 TO 10 BALLS

10 dried pitted dates

½ cup raw walnut halves

½ cup raw pecan halves

¼ cup smooth nut butter

2 tablespoons unsweetened cocoa powder, plus more for rolling if desired

1 tablespoon chia seeds

Unsweetened coconut flakes for rolling (optional)

The secret to these nutty nuggets is that they taste like they're baked, but they're not. They're hearty and portable!

Pulse all ingredients in a food processor until a sticky batter forms.

Kid's job! Scoop 1 to 2 tablespoons of the batter into your hand and roll it into a ball. If desired, place a small amount of cocoa powder and/or coconut flakes on separate pieces of wax paper and roll the ball around in the coating(s) to make it "fluffy." Repeat with the remaining batter.

MOUSE NIBBLES

MAKES 4 TO 5 CUPS

½ cup unsweetened, sulfur-free dried mango slices

¾ cup raw or salted roasted pecans, roughly chopped

¾ cup raw or salted roasted cashews

½ cup salted roasted sunflower seeds

½ cup popped popcorn

Sea salt to taste

We aren't keen on the standard store-bought trail mix that's packed with M&Ms and sugary cranberries. This recipe is easy to make and works as a perfect on-the-go snack. We use raw or roasted nuts without any flavoring or added seasoning, since those usually contain chemicals, sugars, and preservatives. We also use unsweetened, sulfur-free dried fruit. Kids can do every step of this recipe—and they'll be less likely to pick out the jewels when they make it themselves.

Kid's job! Snip, snip. Using child scissors, chop the dried mango into tiny pieces. We like to miniaturize our mango so it provides tiny sweet bursts in every bite of the mix.

Mix the remaining ingredients together in a large bowl. Add the mango and stir.

INVENTORS' CIRCLE

Make Your Own

Here's a template your kids can use to create a protein-packed trail mix. Grown-ups set out the ingredients options in ramekins, and kids choose what goes in. Set out a bunch of nuts and seeds in small dishes, plus one or two dried-fruit options. Kids are welcome to use any or all of the fruits, nuts, and seeds you put out. Name your signature trail mix!

½ cup unsweetened, unsulfured dried fruit: try mango, apricot, apple, or raisins

¾ cup nuts: try pistachios, pecans, cashews, or peanuts

¾ cup nuts: try another kind of nut

¾ cup seeds: try sunflower seeds or pumpkin seeds

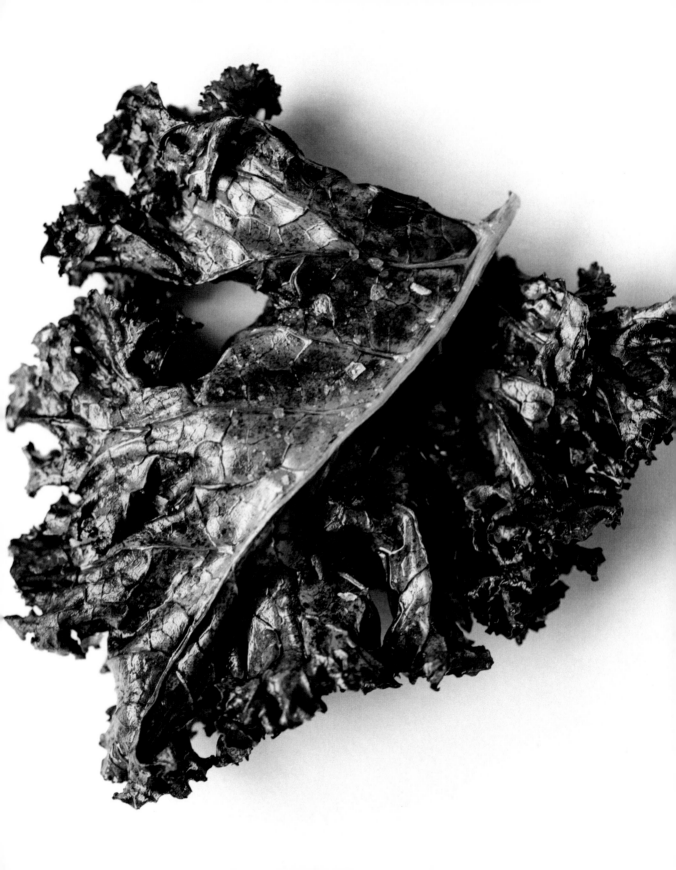

LEAF CHIPS

SERVES 4

1 bunch curly kale
(about 6 cups leaves,
firmly packed)

2 tablespoons olive oil

Sea salt to taste

These chips are so addictive that you may find your family has downed three heads of kale during a single round of battleship. They're as crunchy and satisfying as Doritos, with none of the neon. We find that curly kale crisps best.

Preheat the oven to 300°F.

Kid's job! Prep the leaves by dipping the head of kale in a bowl of cool water. Gently swirl it to remove any dirt. Destem the leaves and tear them into large pieces, each about the size of a gerbil. Now pat dry using a clean towel, or spin the leaves in a salad spinner. Make sure your kale is as dry as possible.

Using your hands, toss the kale in a bowl with the olive oil and salt. Spread the pieces out in a single layer on a baking sheet.

Pop the baking sheet in the oven. Making the chips will take about 10 to 15 minutes. Theoretically, they can be stored in an airtight jar, but they seem to get devoured immediately in our family and never make it to storage.

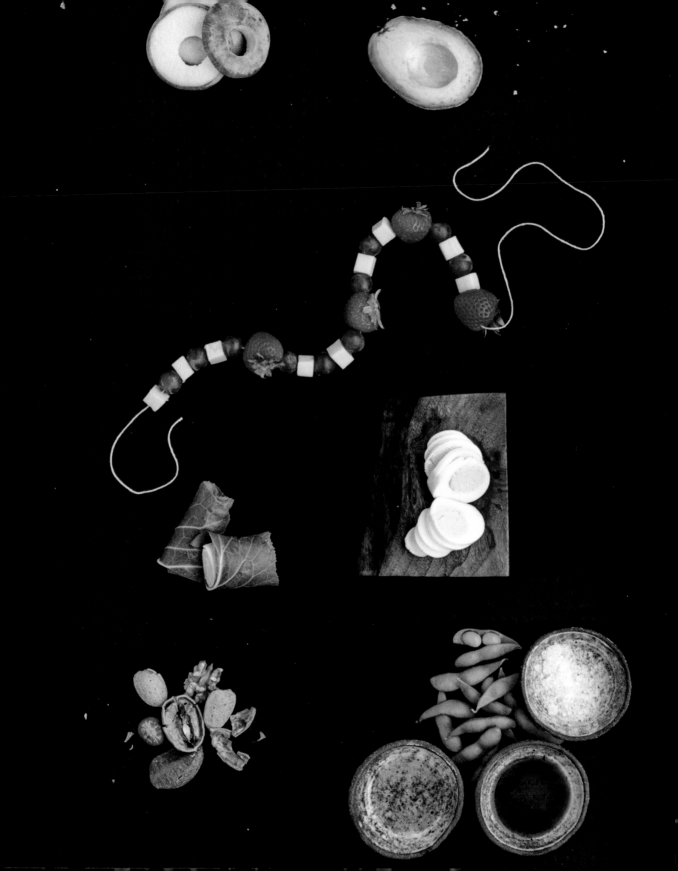

WHOLE-FOOD SNACKS

FOR PARENTS WHO HAVE ZERO TIME

When did squirtable fruit products and crackers become normal snack foods for children? Once we weaned our family off of them, we found that many whole-food snacks are just as easy.

But, but, but. You're thinking, "I need to keep a supply of Goldfish, yogurt in tubes, and Lunchables in the pantry because I'm too busy to make fresh snacks." We get it. We can't spend all day baking protein-packed muffins and cutting them into cute shapes, either. Here's a quick cheat sheet of our family's favorite snack foods for the seriously time challenged. Most take less than three minutes to "prepare." They're rich in protein and fiber because they're actually real foods that haven't been processed into oblivion (please don't blather on about the nutritional value to the kids—they don't care), and kids will dig how much fun they are to prep and eat.

You'll notice that some of these snacks involve deshelling, ripping, smashing, salting, freezing, cutting with kid-safe slicing tools, or rolling—all of which constitute a seriously good time for most kids. Kids also cherish the level of independence they gain from preparing these snacks. Of course, these snacks can be even quicker to prepare if you use preshelled nuts or edamame—we usually prefer to include shells because we've found that the prep process is fun for our children.

Maison's favorite after-school snack: An avocado halved and pitted. She sprinkles on sea salt and a squirt of lemon juice, then eats it with a spoon. (Avocados are tricky to cut safely, so that's the adult's job.)

West's favorite after-school snack: Frozen apple slices.

Turkey Roll: Roll a piece of lettuce or a collard green around a slice of fresh roasted turkey breast.

Squirrel party: Unshelled nuts. Grab a nutcracker or mallet!

Fruit and cheese platter necklace: String some berries, grapes, and cheese together with sturdy craft needles and thread.

Edamame: Let an adult heat some frozen edamame pods, and serve warm. Sprinkle on some sea salt. Rip the pods and pop the little beans into your mouth.

Hard-boiled eggs: Parents, you'll need to boil them. Slice them with an egg slicer. Sprinkle with sea salt.

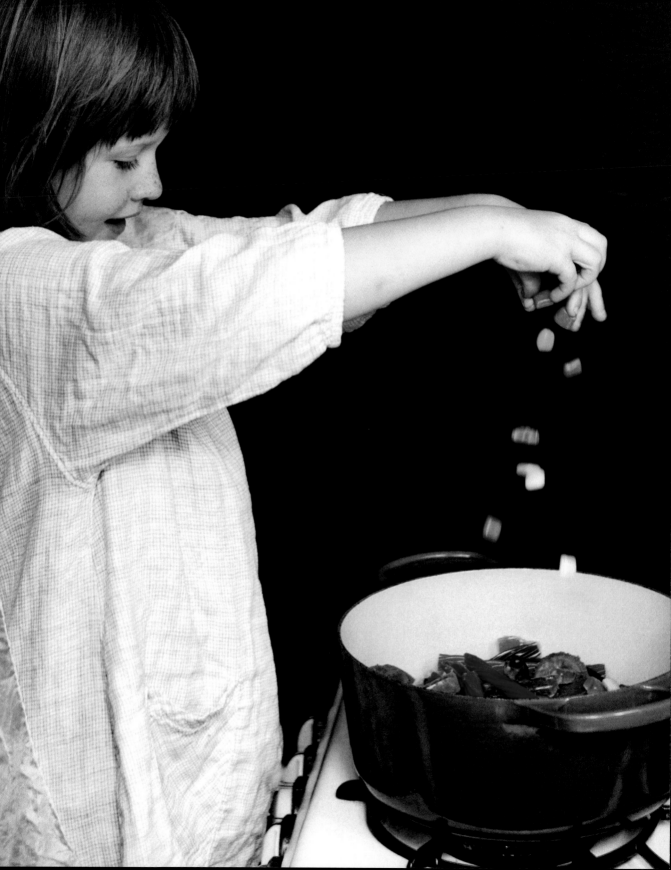

SUGAR
AND SPICE

f your kids are normal human children, they're probably keen on sweets. Zeal for sweets can serve as a gateway to unique new flavors. Sweetness easily works as the bridge between the familiar and the unknown. This chapter features recipes from around the world that give children with limited palates a chance to sample different flavors, textures, and spices.

NOTE: Espresso cups and little dipping bowls are the perfect serving vessels for sweets.

MISHA'S OFFICIAL STATEMENT ON SWEETENERS

What is the best sweetener? This question has been hotly debated. We know that high-fructose corn syrup, saccharine, and NutraSweet aren't recommended for child consumption (or human consumption, for that matter), but what's the "in" sweetener these days? Should we use stevia? Cane sugar? Agave? Honey is definitely delicious, but the very best sweet thing, hands down, is real maple syrup.* You'll notice that the recipes in this chapter rely heavily on real maple syrup.

I grew up in New England, where sugar maples are common. One of my earliest memories is tapping a huge two-hundred-year-old maple tree in our yard, collecting the sap, and boiling it on our stove all day until there was nothing but a sweet, sticky residue at the bottom (aka maple syrup). There are just two weeks every spring when you can harvest sap from sugar maples—the nights have to be below freezing and the days above freezing. That's when the sap begins to flow after the long winter of tree hibernation. In order to make a gallon of maple syrup you have to collect forty gallons of sap and boil it down. While other kids worked at the mall, my after-school job was at a sap house. We used draft horses to pull the wagon that collected the sap. It would take a barnful of wood to boil it down. The smell of the maple steam coming from the giant sap pan, the buds starting to open on the trees, the snow melting in the woods—it all rushes back to me when I taste that delicious combination of minerals and sugars that make up maple syrup.

* When I say maple syrup, I mean 100 percent *real, pure* maple syrup, not the maple-flavored, corn-syrupy stuff some manufacturers try to pass off as maple syrup. I realize some syrup makers consider grade A technically the best, but I prefer grade B—it's so rich and mapley. I also realize real maple syrup is a luxury, but I have such positive childhood associations with it that I can't truly be objective when assessing sweeteners.

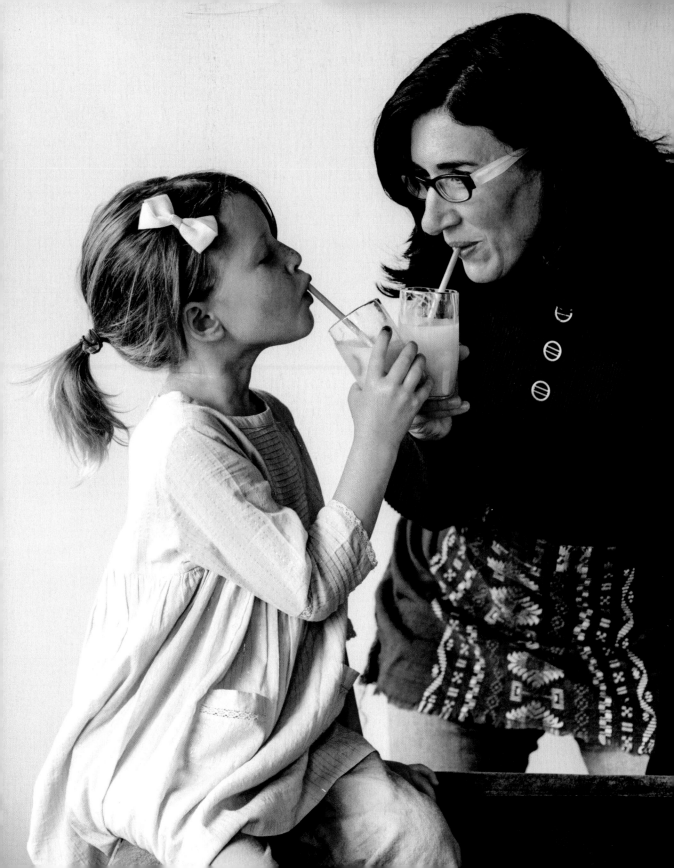

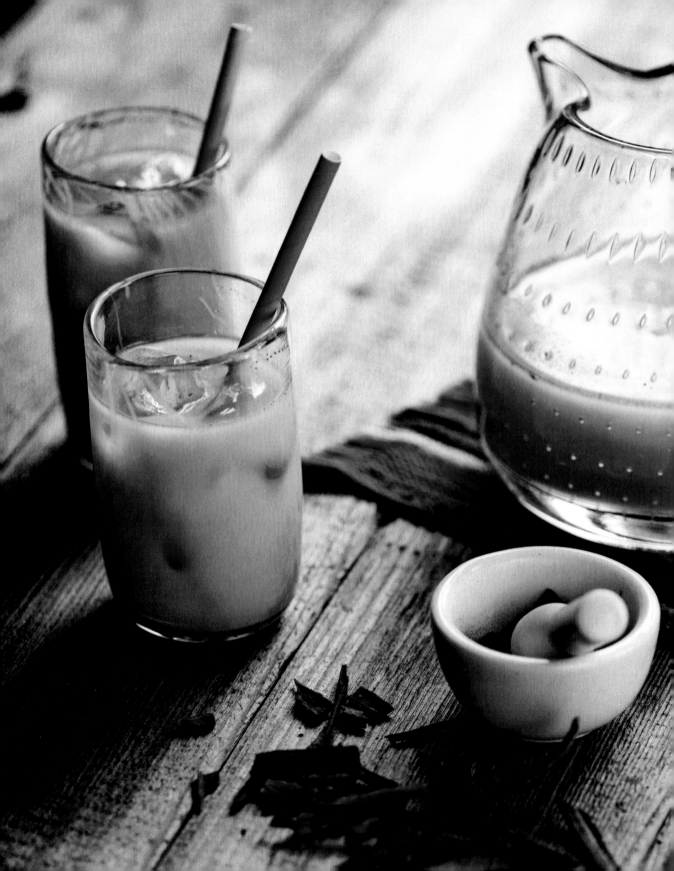

STICK JUICE

SERVES 6 TO 8

I cup uncooked long-grain white rice

4 cinnamon sticks, broken into chunks

I vanilla bean

I tablespoon vanilla extract

I tablespoon maple syrup

5 cups water

Inspired by Mexican horchata, this rice milk is named for the cinnamon sticks that infuse it with flavor. It's easy to make and involves pounding cinnamon sticks, which kids will appreciate. (You'll need some cheesecloth for straining.)

Start by rinsing the rice well in a fine-mesh colander. Pour the cleaned rice into a blender with the remaining ingredients. Blend for 1 minute.

Kid's job! Line a fine-mesh sieve or colander with a double layer of cheesecloth and set it over a pitcher or large bowl. Strain the liquid into the container and serve over ice.

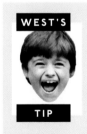

WEST'S

TIP

Use a mortar and pestle or a mallet to smash the cinnamon sticks before dumping them into the blender. A good smashing makes the cinnamon more cinnamony.

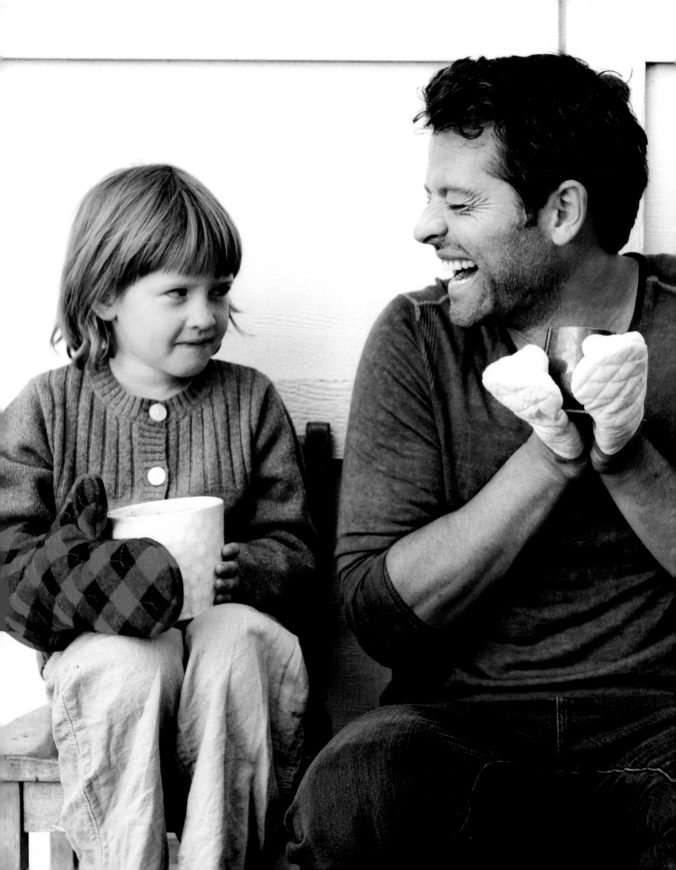

SAY-HELLO-TO-CHILI HOT CHOCOLATE

SERVES 4

2½ cups half-and-half

2 disks (2.7 ounces each) Mexican chocolate (such as Ibarra or Nestlé's Abuelita)

3 cinnamon sticks

¼ dried chile de árbol or pinch of cayenne pepper

Zest of half an orange

Tiny pinch of sea salt

1 vanilla bean

Chocolate shavings for garnish (optional)

Although kids in many parts of the world eat spicy foods, a lot of kids in the US are stuck in the land of the bland. Instead of expecting them to chow down on vindaloo or Szechuan hot pot, we decided to experiment with Mexican hot chocolate, to introduce our children to spice. We drastically reduced the amount of chili in it—and guess what? West sipped and reported, "I even kind of like the spicy part."

Pour your half-and-half into a medium pot and set it over medium heat.

Kid's job! Smashing time: using a mallet, a mortar and pestle, or the smashing implement of your choice, smash your chocolate circles into small chunks and set aside. Then smash the cinnamon sticks and add them to the pot of half-and-half.

Bring the half-and-half mixture to a simmer (don't let it boil) and cook about 5 to 10 minutes, or until nicely cinnamoned. Remove from the heat. Add the chocolate shards to the pot and stir.

Using a mortar and pestle, grind up a teeny-tiny piece of chili (like, pinkie-nail size). Add the powder to the pot along with the orange zest and salt. (Wash your hands after, so you don't accidentally touch your eyes and burn them with chile de árbol flecks.) Whisk until the mixture is smooth and creamy and the chocolate is melted.

Kid's job! Slice open the vanilla bean lengthwise and scrape out the sticky seeds using the side of a butter knife. Throw the seeds and the whole scraped pod into the pot.

continued

Steep 2 minutes longer. Taste. Is it citrusy? Sweet? Does it need more orange zest? Is it spicy? Strain the hot chocolate through a fine-mesh strainer into a pitcher, or cover the top of the pitcher with a double layer of cheesecloth and pour the mixture from the pot into the pitcher.

Pour into tiny espresso cups, top with chocolate shavings if desired, and serve.

ADVENTURE RECIPE

Snow Bowl

Kid's job! When you're tired of playing in the snow, try feasting on it. This is the top-secret recipe that Misha invented when he was a kid growing up in snowy New England.

Fill a small cereal bowl with clean snow. Drizzle with real maple syrup. Add a splash of vanilla extract. Eat with a spoon. When our family is pining for this in the summer, we throw ice cubes in a high-powered blender and blend until we have homemade snow.

LEARNING TO LOVE THE HEAT!

Misha is a hot sauce devotee now, but he still hasn't forgiven the uncle who tricked him into biting into a hot pepper thirty-five years ago. If you want to introduce your kids to spicy foods, prime them first. If you just let them bite into a ghost pepper unawares and unprepared, they're likely to hate you and boycott spices for an eternity. So instead of going for the shock-and-awe strategy, spend some time introducing your kids to aromatic low-heat spices such as garlic, ginger, cinnamon, and nutmeg. Once you've laid the groundwork, add the tiniest drop of hot sauce or fleck of chili pepper to a dish. West and Maison say there's "good spicy" and "bad spicy." (Bad spicy is the kind that makes your face turn red and sweaty.)

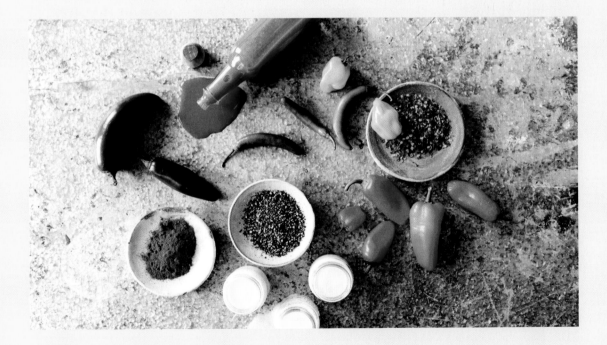

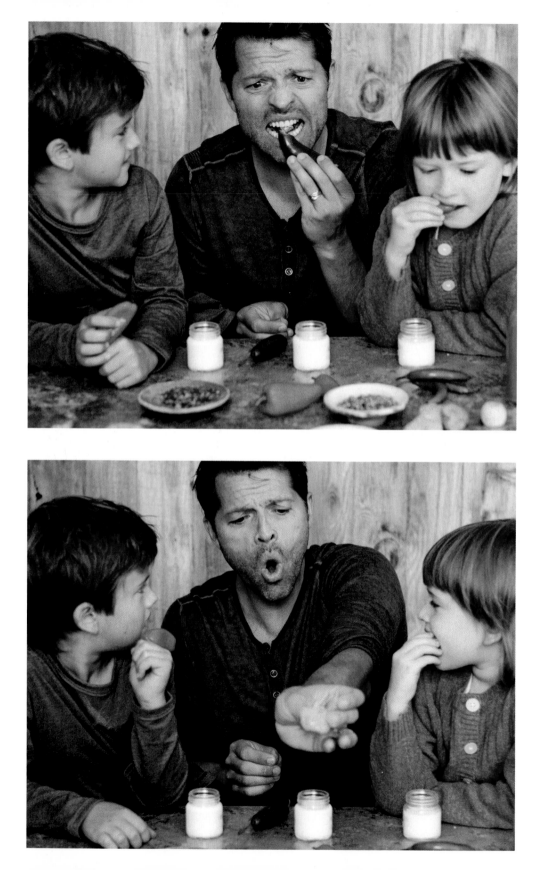

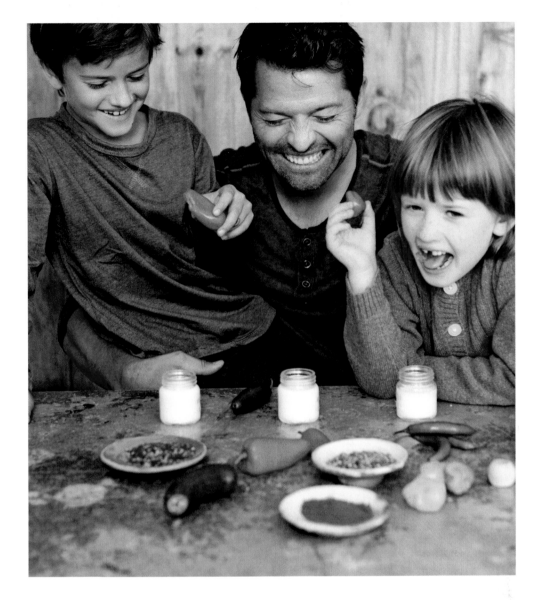

FAMILY CHILI CHALLENGE!

Court danger: Once your kid is willing to flirt with heat, lay out a range of mild to spicy foods and seasonings: paprika, jalapeño peppers, serrano and habanero chilies, hot sauces—and glasses of milk. Try a tiny dot of each one. A lick or maybe even a nibble?

CHOCODILES

FOR BREAKFAST, LUNCH, AND DINNER

The Download on Sugar

What's the scoop on sugar? Is it really the devil? Let us simplify this for you . . . yes and no. (That's really useful, isn't it?) Sugars get absorbed into the body quickly, especially when consumed alone (sans protein), and they cause a quick spike in the concentration of sugar (glucose) in the blood. Sodas, candy, and refined cereals have a high glycemic index, meaning they spike the amount of sugar in your blood rapidly. After the initial hit of energy, blood sugar levels fall below normal range, so kids (and adults) can get moody or feel tired or hungry. Foods that contain fiber, protein, and fat (as opposed to primarily sugar), on the other hand, leave us feeling satisfied longer.

In addition to the blood-sugar roller coaster that leaves us wanting more food, sugar delivers bliss to the entire mouth. Scientists have found taste receptors that light up for sugar all the way down the esophagus to the stomach and pancreas. We're biologically hardwired for sweets. Sugar is so powerful that it can compel us to eat more than we should. Lab rats in one experiment craved sugar so much that it "completely overrode the biological brakes that should have been saying: stop," and within a few weeks of having unlimited sugar access, they ate enough to become obese. Even rats who received electric shocks after eating cheesecake, still lunged for it.

Most parents know that we should consume less sugar. The World Health Organization recommends that all of us, regardless of age, consume less than 10 percent of our daily calories in sugar. This daily intake is easily reached by consuming fruit. The average American adult winds up eating seventy pounds of the stuff a year—four times the recommended amount. Toddlers should max out at four teaspoons of sugar per day, according to the American Heart Association. The average tot in America consumes more than three times that.

In convenience-driven culture, most of the added sugar we consume is hidden in processed food. A study of eight thousand grocery-store foods found that 60 percent of them contain added sugar—including foods you'd never expect to have it, like bologna and stuffing mix. Even foods that don't taste sweet, like pasta sauce and most peanut butters, are loaded with the stuff. "Bread now has sugar in it. Some yogurts have as much sugar as a serving of ice cream," writes Michael Moss, a *New York Times* journalist and the author of *Salt Sugar Fat: How the Food Giants Hooked Us*.

In the quest to make foods consumers crave, food manufacturers have cadres of scientists on staff who specialize in sensory pleasure. They carefully calculate a food's "bliss point" (the precise amount of an ingredient, like sugar or salt, that makes the food most pleasurable) so the manufacturer can concoct just the right ingredient brew for optimal satisfaction.

Food companies are savvy about selling the notion that these convenient kids' foods are healthful, normal, and fun. There's an array of kids' snacks that masquerade as healthful, such as dried fruit (most brands contain added sugar), bottled fruit smoothies (sugar!), flavored yogurt (sugar!), and pretty much anything marketed as a fruit snack (sugar! sugar! sugar!). Parents vastly underestimate the sugar content in these foods, particularly those wearing "health halos," such as yogurt and juice, according to a 2018 study published in the *International Journal of Obesity*.

Food marketing teams employ various strategies for hiding sugar from consumers. A product might list "evaporated cane juice" as one of its ingredients because it sounds more nutritious than sugar—but really, it's just a fancy name for sugar. Food companies employ dozens of other names for sugar, such as agave, barley malt, beet sugar, brown rice syrup, brown sugar, cane sugar, cane syrup, coconut sugar, corn syrup, corn syrup solids, date sugar, dextrin, dextrose, ethyl maltol, fruit juice concentrate, glucose, glucose solids, golden syrup, high-fructose corn syrup, honey, lactose, malt syrup, maltodextrin, maltose, mo-lasses, rice syrup, and sucrose. Food manufacturers often list different *types* of added sugars as the seventh, eighth, and ninth items on an ingredients list to fool us into thinking that the product doesn't contain a significant quantity of added sweeteners. But when you add up all the different types of sweeteners, it makes sugar the number one ingredient.

Sugar in itself isn't evil. There's nothing wrong with enjoying a sweet treat—we devote a chapter to them in this book. It's the daily onslaught of hidden sugars in processed food that throws our relationship with it out of whack. We do our best not to make sugar the "big bad" with our kids. We aren't into making sugar taboo and we aren't into stressing out about it. We just want to keep it in balance, so we try not to let it sneak into their diet in insidious ways. We check the ingredients on packaged foods, and we try to let sweets be an occasional treat instead of the mainstay of their diet. After all, ice cream on a hot summer day is one of the joys of childhood. When West is feeling adventurous, he asks for the weirdest flavor available at our local ice cream shop. Sugar can be a gateway to new flavors and textures.

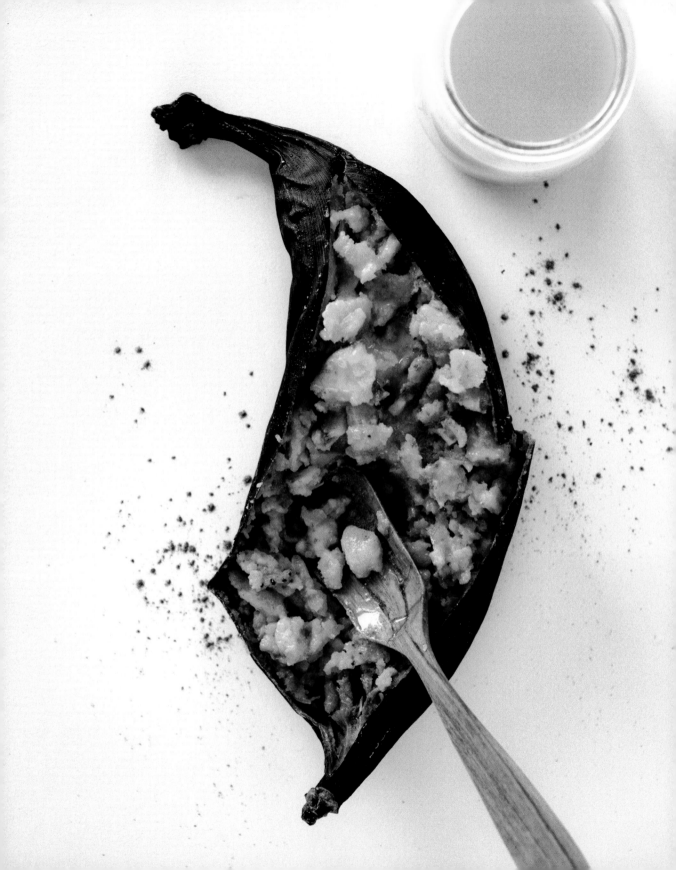

OAXACAN-STYLE GRILLED PLANTAINS

SERVES 4

2 fresh plantains, unpeeled

1 14-ounce can sweetened condensed milk

Cinnamon to taste

The banana's starchier, less sweet cousin, the plantain is a staple of Latin, Caribbean, and African cooking. This recipe is a kid favorite, because that dense banana texture combined with condensed milk and cinnamon makes it taste like warm custard.

Preheat the oven to 350°F.

Put the plantains on a sheet pan lined with parchment paper. Bake for 1 to 1½ hours.

Remove the pan from the oven—the peel will be very black. Let cool a bit before using a sharp knife to cut the skins from top to bottom, just deeply enough to reveal the plantain flesh. Drizzle with condensed milk and sprinkle with cinnamon. Eat with a spoon right out of the peel.

GINGER SPICE COOKIES

MAKES 2 DOZEN
COOKIES

3 cups all-purpose flour

1 teaspoon baking soda

1 teaspoon sea salt

¼ cup powdered ginger

1 cup (2 sticks) butter,
at room temperature

1 cup granulated sugar

1 cup firmly packed
brown sugar

2 eggs

1 tablespoon vanilla
extract

¼ cup grated fresh ginger

¼ cup chopped candied
ginger

Turbinado sugar for
rolling

Misha's aunt used to make these when he was a kid, and we've found that her recipe is an ideal way to explore ginger, which our kids usually find off-puttingly strong. We use three different types of ginger here—powdered, fresh, and candied. This cookie was West's first foray into ginger . . . he said he felt like the cookie bit his tongue, but he kept eating. Now when he tastes ginger in a dish, he doesn't run shrieking from the table. Baby steps.

Preheat the oven to 350°F. Line a baking sheet with parchment paper and set aside.

Kid's job! Start with the dry ingredients. In a large mixing bowl, whisk together flour, baking soda, salt, and powdered ginger. Set aside.

Using an electric mixer—or a wooden spoon, if you are feeling strong—beat together the butter and sugars in a large mixing bowl. Keep beating until the mixture is fluffy and light in color. Add the eggs one at a time, beating well after each addition. Add the vanilla and grated ginger.

Pour half the dry ingredients into the butter mixture and, using a rubber spatula, stir gently until almost all the dry ingredients are mixed in. Then add the remaining dry ingredients, along with the candied ginger, and stir until just incorporated.

Kid's job! Roll your cookie balls. Roll about 2 tablespoons of dough into a ball between your palms and plop it into a dish of turbinado sugar. Give it a good roll around in the sugar, then place it onto your parchment-lined baking sheet. Repeat with the remaining dough, spacing each ball about 2 to 3 inches apart. Press down gently with your palm or the bottom of a glass to flatten each ball.

Bake for 15 minutes. Let them cool in the pan.

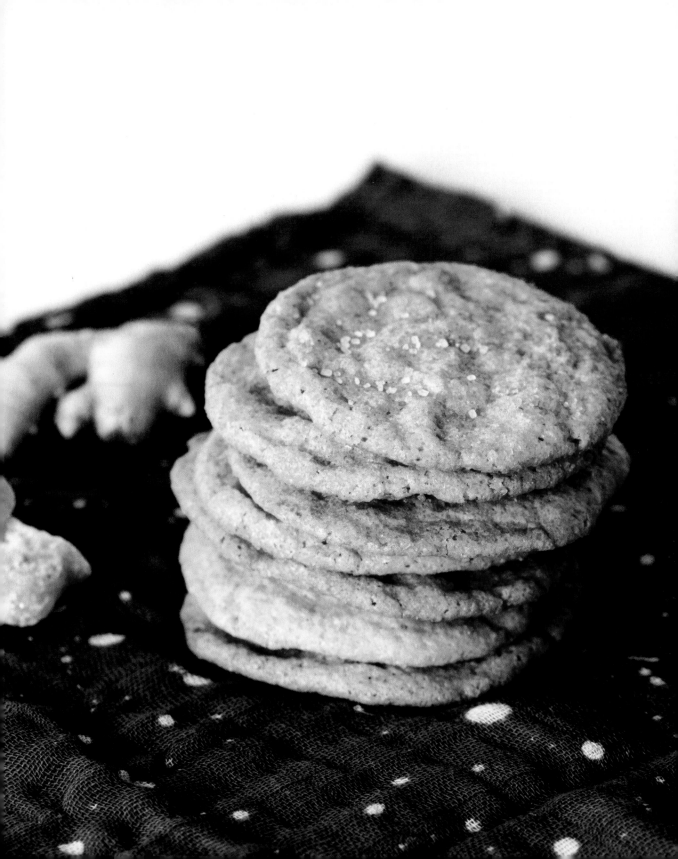

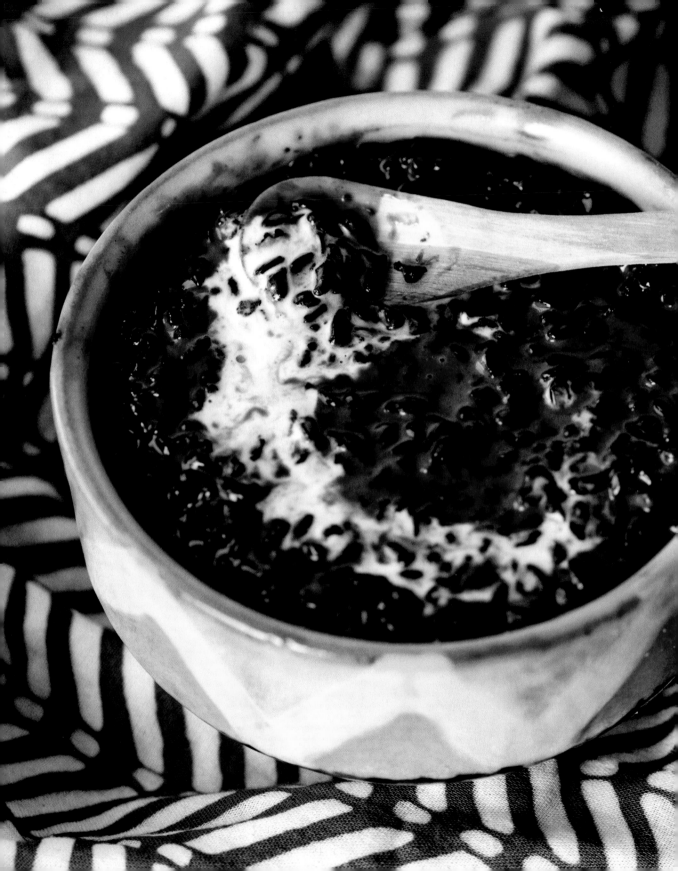

SHOOTING STAR PUDDING

SERVES 4 TO 6

1 cup black rice, soaked in water for a few hours

2 cups water

1½ cups coconut milk

2 cinnamon sticks

2 to 5 whole star anise

½ cup maple syrup

Generous pinch of sea salt

Traditional rice pudding is gloppy, white, and studded with raisins. By contrast, this one is made with black rice, traditionally used in Indian and Thai desserts. In addition to being more glamorous than the traditional version, this pudding contains star anise, which might be a novel flavor for your kids. Another perk of this dish is that it gives kids a chance to eat a familiar food (rice) in a totally different presentation.

Drain and rinse the rice a few times in a fine-mesh colander.

Combine the rice and 2 cups water in a medium pot. Cover, bring to a boil, then turn the heat down and simmer for 45 minutes.

Add the coconut milk, cinnamon, star anise, maple syrup, and salt. Stir and simmer an additional 30 minutes, taking the lid off for the last 10 minutes and stirring occasionally. Spoon into bowls, and serve warm. Don't eat the star anise. But if you find one in your bowl, you get to make a wish!

Adventure Recipe
FRUITY FRONTIERS

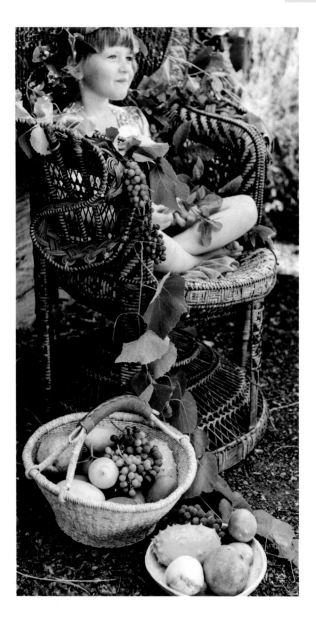

Fruit isn't exactly a tough sell for kids. Since many kids eat fruit willingly, tasting a new one can be a fun family adventure that'll pique everyone's interest.

Kid's job! Go to a grocery store or farmers' market and choose some fruit you've never tasted before. Dragon fruit? Passion fruit? Now make a fruit salad!

Record your tasting adventures! Keep adding to the list.

ROSY RICE PUDDING

SERVES 4 TO 6

1 cup basmati rice

2½ cups water

½ teaspoon sea salt

1 13.6-ounce can coconut milk

1 cup half-and-half

6 tablespoons honey

½ teaspoon rose water

Edible flowers are one of the prettiest ways to expand your kids' palates. Nasturtium, zucchini flowers, and honeysuckle all have unusual flavors without being too strong for kids who are used to bland foods. Rose water, which can be found in the international food section at most grocery stores, adds a delicate flavor.

Rinse the rice a few times in a fine-mesh colander.

Combine the rice, water, and salt in a medium pot and cover. Bring to a boil, then reduce heat to low. Simmer for 20 minutes, then remove from heat and let stand, covered, for 10 minutes.

Add the coconut milk, half-and-half, and honey, then return to a boil over medium heat. Reduce heat to low and cook, stirring frequently, for about 15 to 20 minutes, or until the pudding is creamy. Stir in the rose water and cook for a few minutes more. Serve warm, at room temperature, or chilled.

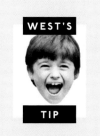

WEST'S

TIP

Sprinkle dandelion flowers or rose petals on top—NOT RAISINS!

IS THERE ANYTHING MISHA WON'T PUT RAISINS ON?

Forget the rose petals—sprinkle raisins on top. After all, raisins make every dish taste better.

RECIPES ONLY A KID COULD DREAM UP

Halloween Candy Stew Freeze

Desperate to thwart our toddler's attempts to consume an entire mountain of Halloween candy, we gave her permission to boil her candy into a stew. The result was so sufficiently unappealing that she stopped eating after one bite.

Kid's job! **Candy dump: unwrap all Halloween candy. Dump it into a large pot—yes, the fruity stuff; yes, the chewy stuff; yes, the chocolatey stuff, the hard candies, the minty candies.**

Melt it down. Heat the mixture over medium heat, stirring frequently. Watch the candies bubble, curdle, melt, and dissolve. Once you have a sludgy brown goo, it's ready. It should be uneven and lumpy. Remove the pot from the heat. Let it cool for a few minutes.

Freeze it. Pour the mixture onto a cookie sheet and freeze for at least several hours. Do not cover—this will ensure freezer burn. When the mixture is solid, it's ready to nibble and discard.

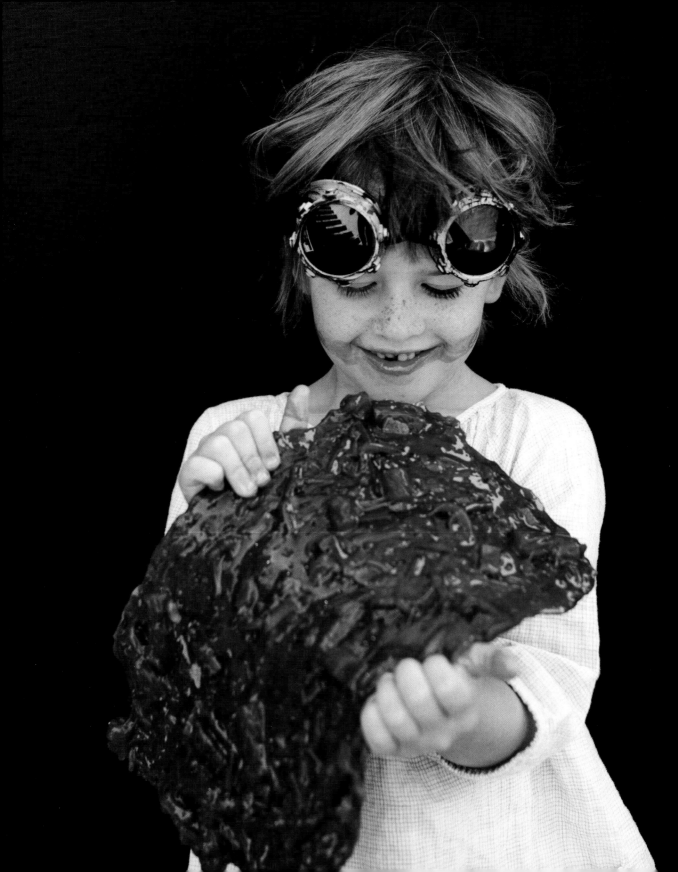

MY KID EATS

ONLY **MUFFINS, OREOS,** AND **FROOT LOOPS, OH, MY!**

Pretty much everyone on the planet knows that sugar is easy to love. It's delicious. If your family generally eats whole foods, adding a dessert here and there can easily be cataloged as one of the joys of family life. In American culture, however, most kids' diets are already packed with sugar from all the processed foods they eat. That's when sugar consumption gets out of whack. Sugar isn't automatically a bad thing. We're not jumping onto the sugar-is-the-devil bandwagon—we all probably realize too much sugar isn't great for us. So if it's sugar, sugar, sugar all day long, and you're itching to change your family's eating habits, kids'-food experts have some strategies for you to consider.

Read the Ingredients

Since food manufacturers go to great lengths to sneak sugar into processed foods by renaming it, you probably don't know how much of the stuff your family is consuming. One way to find out is to read the ingredients lists. Did you know that every time your kid downs a flavored yogurt she's getting nearly her entire recommended daily sugar allowance at once? Becoming aware of the sneaky sugars—particularly in snack foods designed for kids—can be really helpful.

Don't Make Sweets Taboo

Internationally renowned child-food expert Ellyn Satter suggests a few approaches to sugar. She's firm in her belief that no food should be totally off-limits for kids. "Don't make sweets the forbidden fruit," says Satter. "If you do, kids will overeat when given them." Making a food taboo tends to ramp up kids' desire for it.

Stop making such a stink about sweets. Chances are, if you're American, you feel conflicted about sugar. Sometimes you crave it, yet you feel guilty when you eat a piece of cake. Try not to pass your own inner sugar turmoil on to your kids. Remember: negative attention draws interest. Instead of making a big deal about the cookie your kid just ate, let him eat it, savor every morsel of it, and be done with it. We hype up goodies as "bad" and tightly control them. "There's nothing wrong with sweets! Be neutral about goodies and avoid giving them added attention. Send the message that sweets are a nice part of life and not something to feel guilty about," says pediatric food therapist Maryann Jacobsen.

Neutralize the power of goodies.

STRATEGY 1: STOP USING SWEETS TO REWARD AND BRIBE

How many times have you said, "Eat your vegetables and you can have dessert?" Cut it out. It's tempting to hold out the promise of dessert as a reward for good behavior or for eating veggies, but research shows that using sweets as a reward or bribe intensifies kids' desire for sweet foods and increases their dislike of the "have-to-eat" foods.

STRATEGY 2:
SERVE DESSERT WITH DINNER (YEAH, YOU READ THAT RIGHT)

Make dessert part of your family dinner occasionally. Serving a sliver of brownie on your kid's dinner plate normalizes the concept and strips sweets of their power. Tiny portions also emphasize how much sweet stuff your kid should be eating—without you having to say much about it. Let your kid eat the sweet whenever she wants during the meal. Yep, that means she could choose to eat dessert first. It's a single serving—one wee portion. No seconds. If your kid whines about wanting more, try: "If you're hungry, you can have some of the other food on your plate, like the potatoes, peas, and chicken."

STRATEGY 3:
DEVELOP A FAMILY SWEETS POLICY

If sweets have become a big thing in your house, and you're annoyed by frequent negotiations, kids'-food experts suggest that parents develop a family policy. Make sure it's one you can stick to. Let the kids know the plan, then don't waver. The upside: if you adhere to the plan, your kids will eventually stop trying to negotiate more sweets, and you'll all be more relaxed.

For example, let your children choose one sweet per day or one sweet per week (for example, a waffle with maple syrup, a muffin, or ice cream). What plan works best for your family? Parents, develop the plan on your own, then tell your kids.

Write down your family sweets plan.

STRATEGY 4:
UNLIMITED SWEETS

Have you ever heard of Lördagsgodis? It's a Swedish tradition that calls for children and adults to eat as many sweets as they want, but only one day a week. The rest of the week, it's zero sweets. (Translated roughly, it means "Saturday candy.") Some American kids'-food experts agree with this approach. The upside, it eliminates the terror of sugar scarcity. *(No gummy bears ever???!!)*

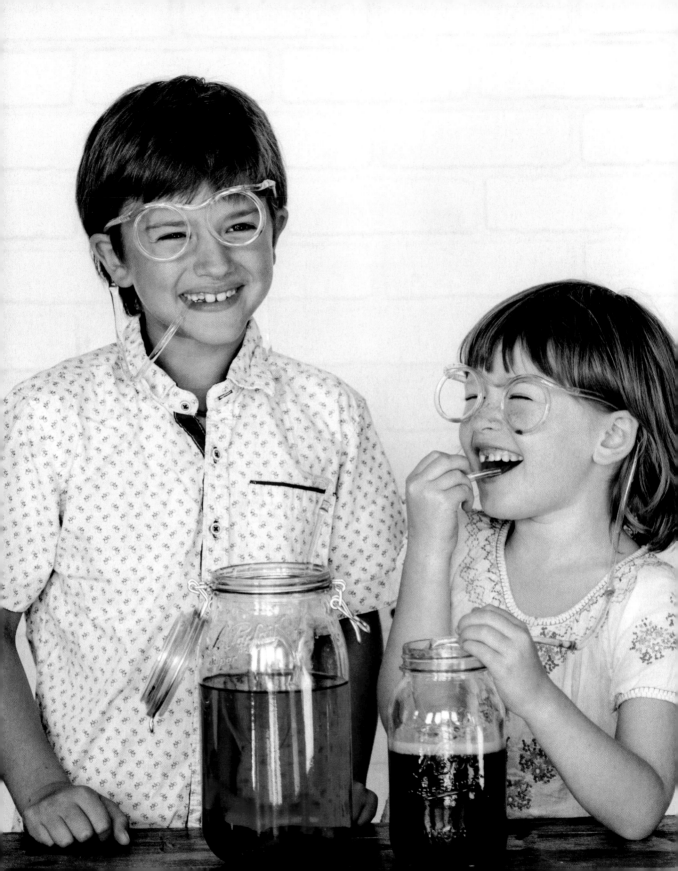

DARING
AND
DELICIOUS
DRINKS

Medical professionals have been urging parents to serve kids fewer sugary drinks for decades. But between 2011 and 2014, about two-thirds of children in the US consumed at least one sweetened drink on any given day, and roughly 30 percent consumed two or more per day. These drinks include lemonade, sports drinks, sweetened iced tea, sodas, and fruit punch, which have been linked to long-term weight gain and a host of health issues, including diabetes.

Turns out, the perfect drink for kids is . . . drumroll, please . . . water. But if you're in the mood for something more exotic, here are our family's other favorite liquid inventions—playful homemade juices, nut milks, teas, and waters with a twist—to give you some alternatives to colas and lemonades without sucking the fun out of hydration.

MISHA'S SUGAR FIX: When I was nine years old, I got a newspaper route, which put spending money in my pocket for the first time. Every week, I had twenty-five bucks to spend on whatever I wanted—and what I wanted was junk food. I'd take my little brother to the Inkwell News convenience store and we'd load up on Hostess Fruit Pies, Mountain Dew, Doritos, Chocodiles, Charleston Chews, and every other artificially colored, corn-syrupy morsel we could get our hands on. My favorite drinks were Yoo-hoo, Capri Sun, Dr Pepper, and Juicy Juice. We also got Crystal Light for free from our local food pantry, which was a huge score, in my opinion. I'm not sure why these drinks were ever approved by the FDA or why anyone ever considered it appropriate to serve these to kids, but let me tell you, I found them deeeelicious. I'm not sure if it was the Doritos or the Yoo-hoos, but I spent more and more time on the couch, and within two years, I had gained twenty pounds. By the time I was eleven, I was depressed.

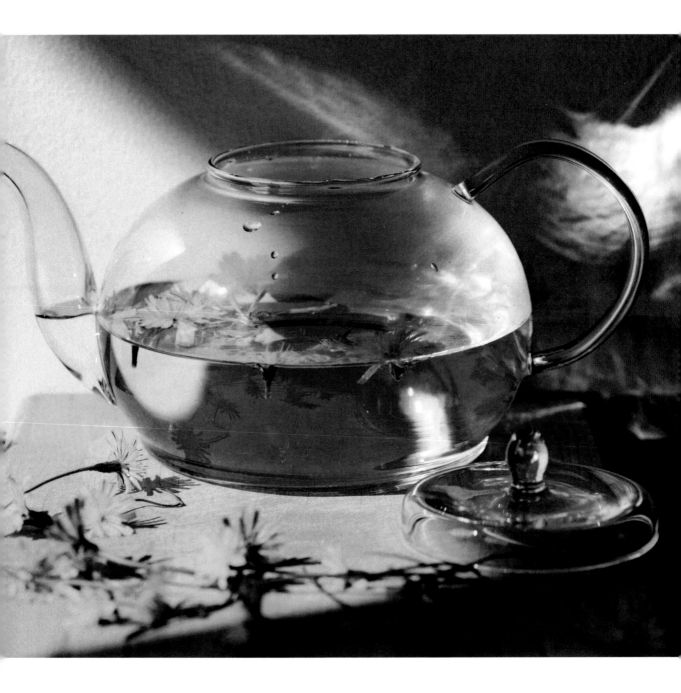

T-SHIRT TEA

SERVES 4

10 whole cloves

8 cardamom pods

2 cinnamon sticks

Pinch of grated fresh ginger (if your kid is feeling brave)

4 cups cold water

2 rooibos tea bags

1 cup milk

Honey to taste

Splash of vanilla extract

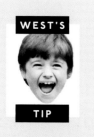

WEST'S

TIP

While you're counting out all these new and fun spices, give each one a sniff. Does the smell get stronger or weaker after you smash them? When you're done crushing, wear your spice-smashing T-shirt around: instant perfume.

Grown-ups like this caffeine-free chai recipe because it gives kids an opportunity to smell and touch a bunch of spices. Kids like this recipe because they get to smash and obliterate the spices with a mallet. We do this in our garage for easier cleanup. A note about spices: we like to stock up on spices in the bulk-foods section of the health food store or local food co-op (it's thriftier than those tiny jars in the baking section of the supermarket). Other spots where you can score chai spices: Indian or Asian grocery stores.

Kid's job! Lay out an old T-shirt on the floor. Place the cloves, cardamom pods, and cinnamon sticks in a small pile on top of your T-shirt. Now wrap the edges of your shirt over the spices. Put on some goggles to protect your eyes. These spices can fly. Using the smashing instrument of your choice, smash the spices. When spices are crushed to your satisfaction, set aside and grate some ginger.

Pour the cloves, cardamom, and cinnamon out of the T-shirt and into a medium pot. Add the water and bring to a boil over high heat. Add ginger and reduce the heat to medium-low and simmer gently for 10 minutes. Remove from heat. Add the tea bags and steep, covered, for 5 minutes. Discard the tea bags.

Sweeten it up: add milk, honey, and vanilla. Bring the tea back to a simmer over high heat, stirring until the honey dissolves. Strain with a fine-mesh strainer into a teapot and serve hot, or let it cool and pour over ice.

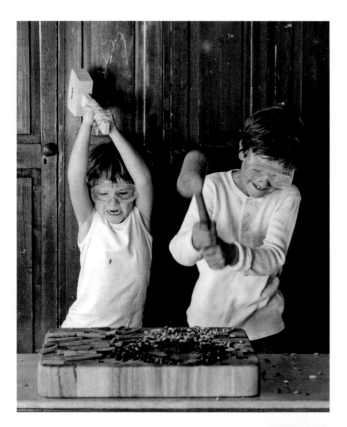

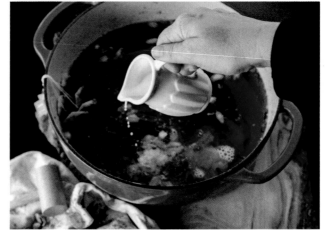

MISHA'S TIP

Chai is usually made with caffeinated tea. Our kids definitely don't need more energy, so we use rooibos tea as the base—it's a mellow, sweetly flavored herbal tea that's darn delicious in chai, and kids love it. For adults who want an added kick, separate out some of the hot water and use regular black tea.

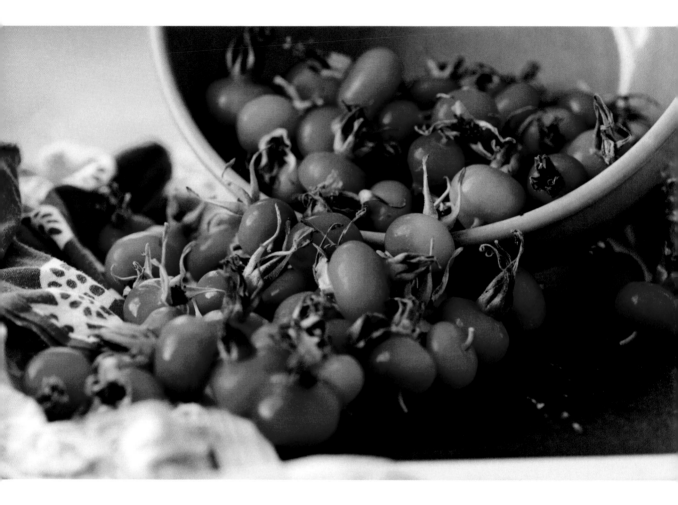

Adventure Recipe

HANDPICKED WILD ROSE HIPS TEA

SERVES 4 TO 6

Handful of foraged rose hips

5 cups water

Ever notice those little red-orange fruits growing on rosebushes after the flowers fall off? Those ubiquitous little gems are called rose hips. They're edible and can be eaten raw or cooked. They have a tartness that West and Maison love. Avoid the hairs inside the fruit, which can tickle your throat. We like to use rose hips to make a hot winter tea, and they're packed with vitamin C. (Fun fact: rose petals are also edible.)

Kid's job! Collect, wash, dry, and smash.

Walk around your neighborhood foraging for rose hips—wild rosebushes are common in abandoned lots and parks all over. Collect as many as you'd like. Chuck any smooshed or rotten ones.

Wash the rose hips in a colander under cold running water, then pat them dry with a towel. String them together with a needle and thread, then hang your rose-hip garland in the sun to dry. It could take up to three sunny days. You'll know they're done when they're hard, dark brown, leathery, and wrinkled.

Once the fruits have dried, pluck off the stalks and the little pointy pricks at the top. Put the trimmed rose hips in a large zip-lock bag and smash them with a mallet. Don't grind them too small. Now pour the rose-hip powder through a sieve. This should help remove the tiny hairs that can tickle your throat.

Bring the water to a boil in a medium pot over high heat. Put one or two teaspoons of rose-hip powder into a teapot, then fill with boiling water. Let sit for 15 to 20 minutes. Strain. Drink.

Save your extra rose-hip powder in a jar with a tight-fitting lid.

NUTTY MILK

SERVES 4 TO 6

2 cups raw unsalted almonds

4 cups water

I teaspoon vanilla extract

2 dried pitted dates

Pinch of cinnamon

Pinch of sea salt

Nut milk is a protein-packed, creamy wonder drink. It's ridiculously easy to make if you have a powerful blender, which we recommend you use to make this drink. Many prepackaged nut milks contain added preservatives—our homemade version only contains the good stuff. You'll need cheesecloth.

Put the almonds in a bowl and add enough water to cover. Let sit at room temperature for at least an hour, preferably overnight. Drain and rinse, discarding the soaking water. Put the soaked nuts in a powerful blender, then add the 4 cups water, vanilla, dates, cinnamon, and salt.

Kid's job! Be the timer: when your grown-up starts the blender, start singing the alphabet. When you're done singing, the blending is done!

Kid's job! Get your squeeze on! Now you'll need to strain the milk. Using a clean piece of cheesecloth, cover the top of a large bowl. Start pouring the nut milk through the cloth into the bowl. When the fabric has a nice chunk of nut mush in it, squeeze it tight to let the liquid drip through. Give it another good squeeze and a squish.

Once you've strained all the milk, start sipping. Try pouring it over your favorite cereal or in your smoothies. It'll last five days in the fridge.

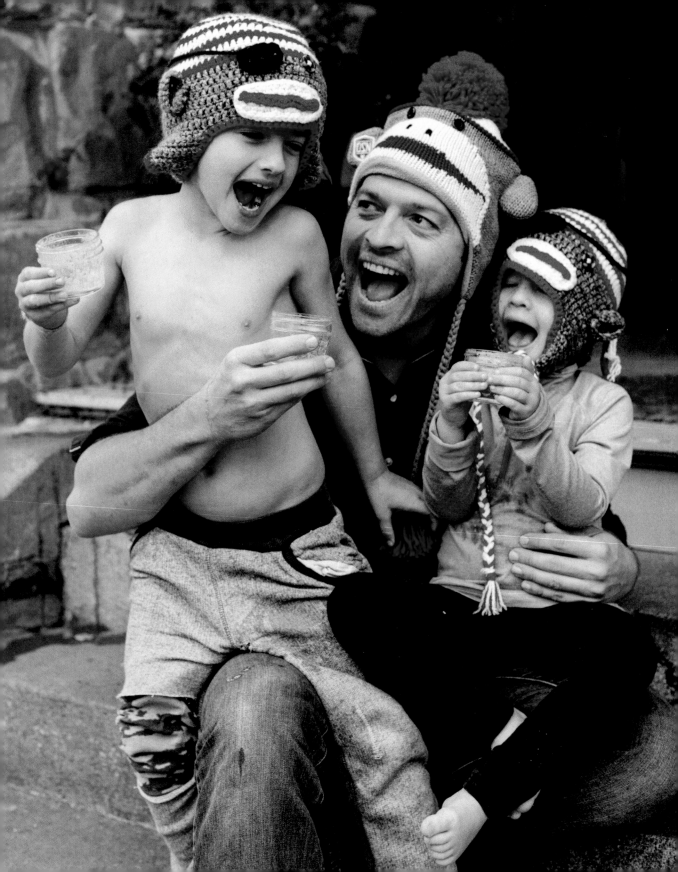

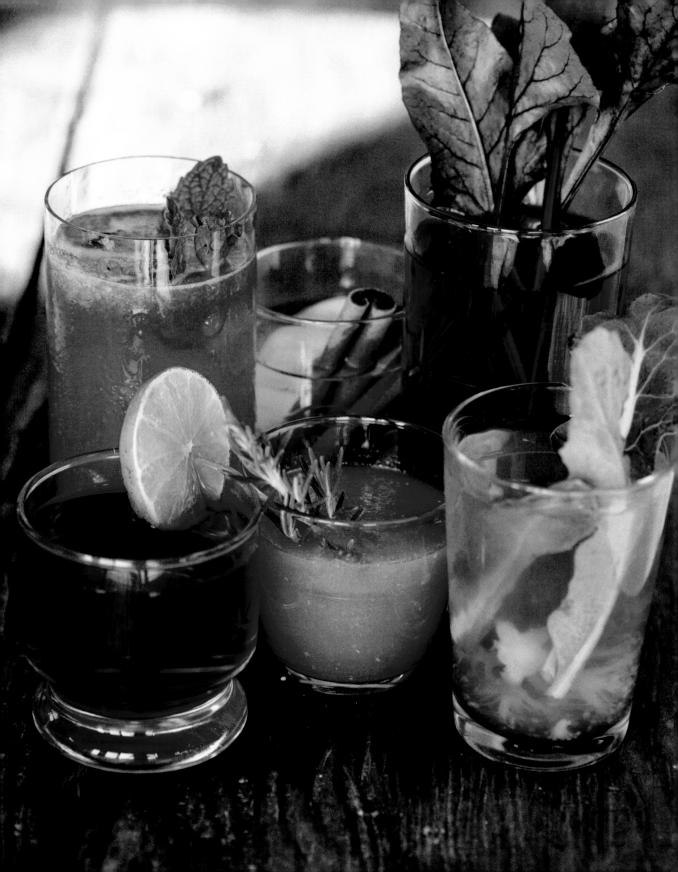

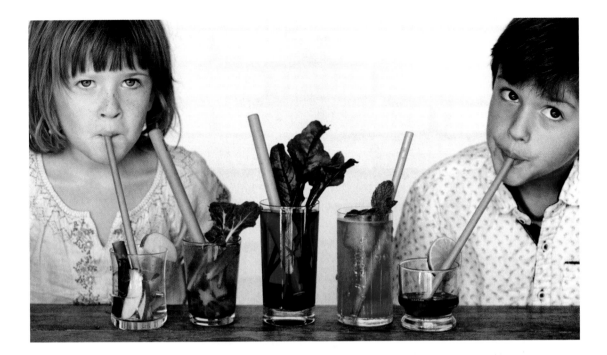

SPLASH-FREE FUN WITH WATER!

Did you know that our bodies are made mostly of water? Water makes you faster, smarter, stronger, and more fun. Even though water is perfect as it is, we like to invent new waters. (Ask a grown-up to help with anything that requires boiling or blending. The rest is up to you.)

Pink ice: Throw some fresh seeded watermelon chunks in the blender with a cup of water. Blend the mixture into an ice cube tray. Freeze. Build a tower of pink ice inside your glass of water.

Pink water: Throw a slice of raw beet into a glass of water. Watch it turn fuchsia.

Broccoli water: Yep, you read that right. This is an unexpected favorite in our house. Pour the leftover water from cooking broccoli into drinking glasses—it's warm, salty, delightfully green, and strangely tasty. Sample it. What do you think?

Mouth-pucker water: Pour a few spoonfuls of unsweetened cranberry juice (make sure it contains no added grape or apple juice or sweeteners) into a glass of water. Serve it to your parents and friends. Who puckers up when they take a swig? Can you invent another water that makes your mouth pucker?

Flower power tea: Pick some dandelions. Wash them. Throw the yellow petals in hot water. Drain and pour into teacups. Drink. Does the color yellow have a flavor?

Raindrop tea: Whenever it rains, Maison runs straight outside to feel every drop. "I just love everything outside," Maison says. "I love rain. I love snow. I love wind." She invented her own recipe for raindrop tea: set some bowls outside in the rain. Let them collect rainwater. Then warm the water in a pot. Pour it into teacups. Sip. Can you taste thunder and lightning?

WATERMELON-LIME JUICE

SERVES 2 TO 3

1 cup water

4 cups seedless
watermelon chunks

Juice of 1 lime

Sprig of mint (optional)

Have you ever made fresh watermelon juice on a hot summer day? This glorious juice is a required summer treat for our family.

Combine watermelon chunks, water, and lime juice in a high-powered blender. Blend until frothy pink and smooth. Serve over ice and garnish with a sprig of mint if desired.

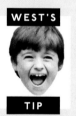

WEST'S

TIP

Some people eat watermelon with a little salt. Salted watermelon is a popular tradition in Japan. Feeling adventurous? Go ahead—sprinkle a little sea salt on your watermelon.

WATERMELON: FRUIT OR VEG?

Let's start with a highly controversial question: is watermelon a fruit or a vegetable? Believe it or not, this beloved pink food suffers an identity crisis. Botanists designate it a fruit, but Oklahoma officially designated it the state vegetable in 2007. Watermelon is part of the cucumber family—the most delicious member, if you ask us—and it grows on a vine, as vegetables do. In some culinary circles, it's even treated as a vegetable.

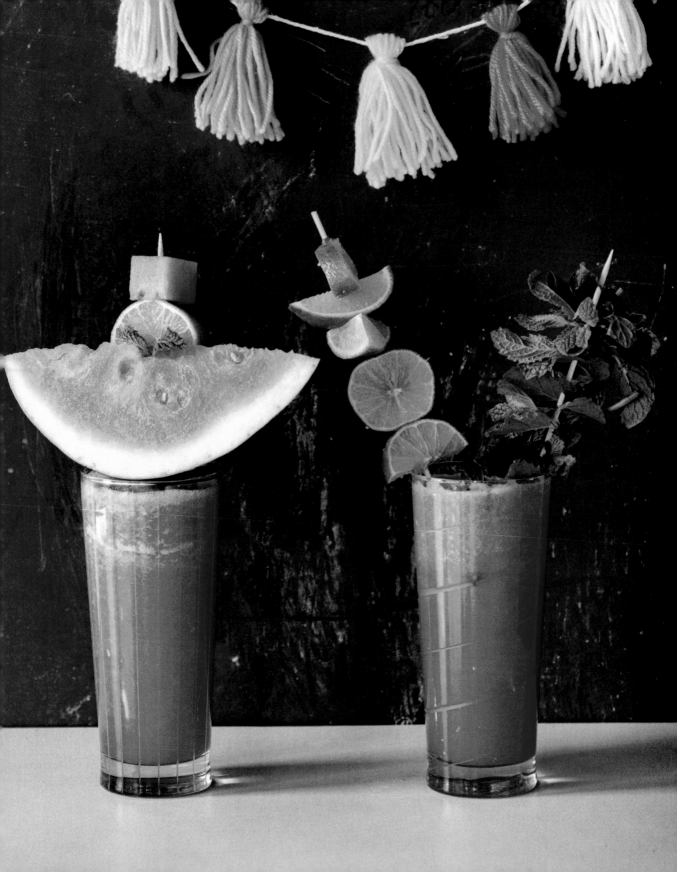

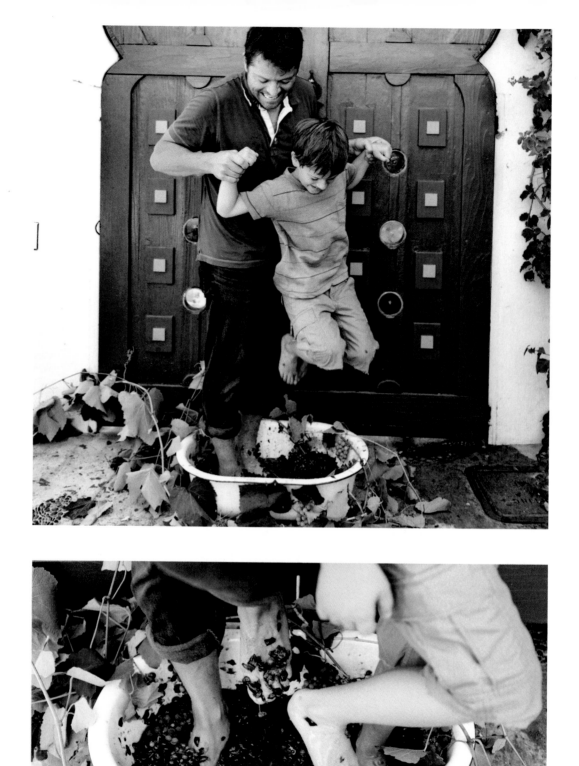

Adventure Recipe

GRAPE STOMP JUICE

SERVES 8 TO 10

4 to 5 bunches grapes, around 5 pounds

Have you ever heard the golden rule of cooking—don't step in your food? Encourage your children to break that rule. You'll need a strainer and one extra-large bucket.

Kid's job! Pluck those stems off the grapes. Make sure to get every little piece of stem off. Throw the destemmed grapes into the large bucket.

Clean those toes: remove your shoes and wash your feet with warm water and soap.

Next, step directly into the extra-large bucket filled with grapes. On the way, don't step on any grass or anything else. Now that you're ankle deep in grapes, stomp to your heart's content. Stomp until you've mashed your grapes into purple puddles.

When you're finished stomping grapes, rinse your feet with a garden hose. Bring a fine-mesh colander or sieve outside, scoop your pulpy grape mush into it, and strain the juice into a large pot. This will filter out the skin, seeds, and pulp.

Bring the filtered juice to a boil over high heat and let it simmer for 10 minutes to heat out any germs. Let it cool, then pour over ice and drink.

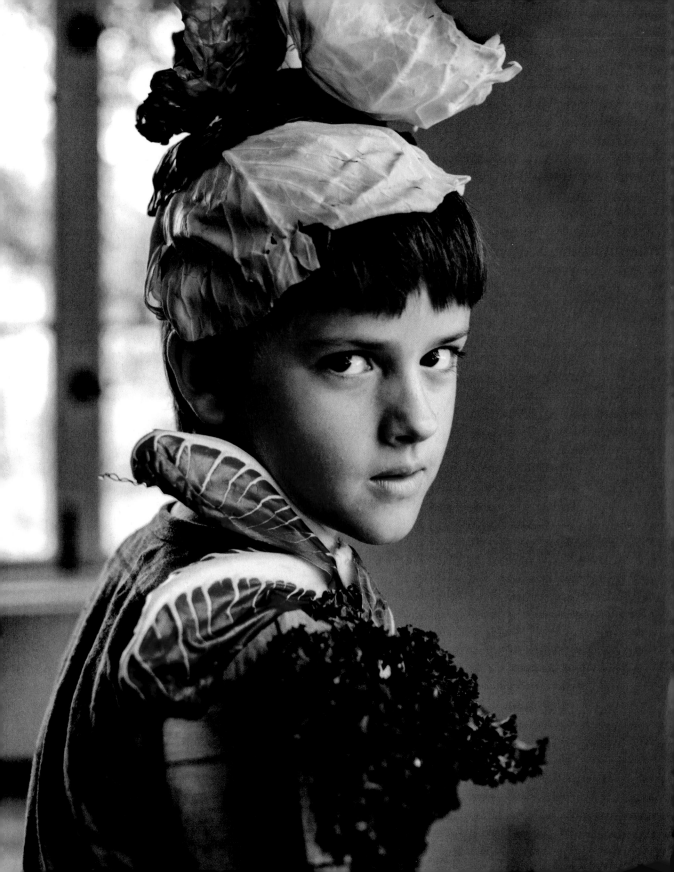

RESOURCES FOR YOUNG EATERS

For more resources, visit www.adventurouseatersclub.com.

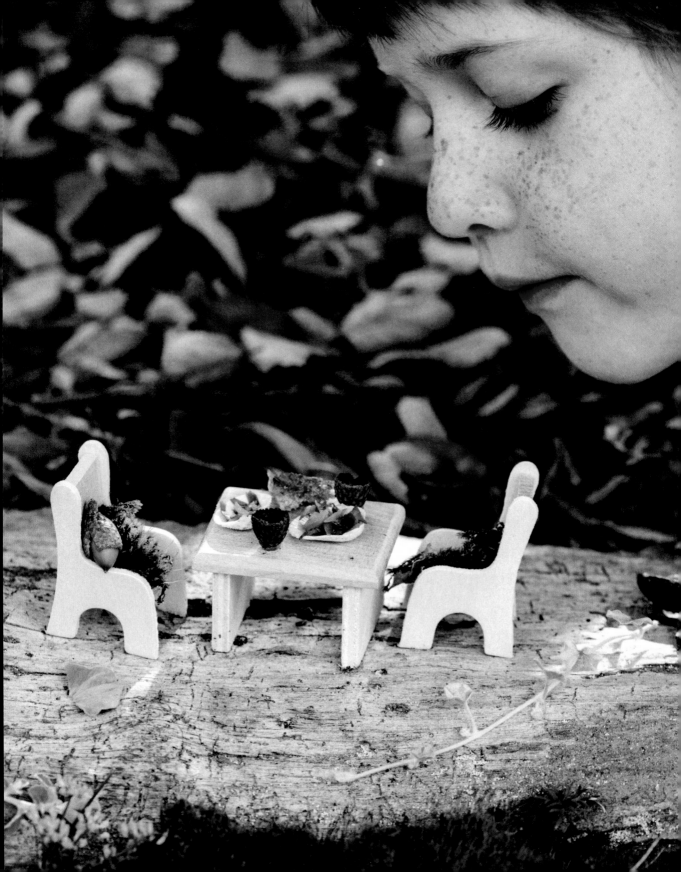

ADVENTUROUS READING LIST

Gardening and Foraging

All New Square Foot Gardening: The Revolutionary Way to Grow More in Less Space, 2nd ed., by Mel Bartholomew (Minneapolis, MN: Cool Springs Press, 2013).

Rocks, Dirt, Worms & Weeds: A Fun, User-Friendly, Illustrated Guide to Creating a Vegetable or Flower Garden with Your Kids by Jeff Hutton (New York: Skyhorse Publishing, 2012).

From Seed to Skillet: A Guide to Growing, Tending, Harvesting, and Cooking Up Fresh, Healthful Food to Share with People You Love by Jimmy Williams and Susan Heeger (San Francisco: Chronicle Books, 2010).

Backyard Foraging: 65 Familiar Plants You Didn't Know You Could Eat by Ellen Zachos (North Adams, MA: Storey Publishing, 2013).

Music

Dancing in the Kitchen: Songs That Celebrate the Joy of Food! by Joan Huntsberry Langford, at store.cdbaby.com

Expert (and Nonexpert) Wisdom on Kids and Food

Adventures in Veggieland: Help Your Kids Learn to Love Vegetables with 100 Easy Activities and Recipes by Melanie Potock, MA, CCC-SLP (New York: The Experiment, 2018).

The Yale Guide to Children's Nutrition by William V. Tamborlane, MD (New Haven, CT: Yale Univ. Press, 1997).

Food Love Family: A Practical Guide to Child Nutrition by Maya Adam (San Diego, CA: Cognella Academic Publishing, 2016).

From Picky to Powerful: The Mindset, Strategies, and Know-How You Need to Empower Your Picky Eater by Maryann Jacobsen, MS, RD (RMI Books, 2016).

How to Raise a Mindful Eater: 8 Powerful Principles for Transforming Your Child's Relationship with Food by Maryann Jacobsen, MS, RD (RMI Books, 2016).

Nutrition: What Every Parent Needs to Know, 2nd ed., by William H. Diets, MD, PhD, FAAP, and Loraine Stern, MD, FAAP (Itasca, IL: American Academy of Pediatrics, 2012).

Helping Your Child with Extreme Picky Eating: A Step-by-Step Guide for Overcoming Selective Eating, Food Aversion, and Feeding Disorders by Katja Rowell, MD, and Jenny McGlothlin, MS, SLP (Oakland, CA: New Harbinger Publications, 2015).

Raising a Healthy, Happy Eater: A Stage-by-Stage Guide to Setting Your Child on the Path to Adventurous Eating by Nimali Fernando, MD, MPH, and Melanie Potock, MA, CCC-SLP (New York: The Experiment, 2015).

Bringing Up Bébé: One American Mother Discovers the Wisdom of French Parenting by Pamela Druckerman (New York: Penguin Press, 2012).

The Languages of Food: Recipes, Experiences, Thoughts edited by Ilaria Cavallini and Maddalena Tedeschi (Reggio Emilia, Italy: Reggio Children, 2008).

First Bite: How We Learn to Eat by Bee Wilson (New York: Basic Books, 2015).

French Kids Eat Everything: How Our Family Moved to France, Cured Picky Eating, Banned Snacking, and Discovered 10 Simple Rules for Raising Happy, Healthy Eaters by Karen Le Billon (New York: William Morrow, 2012).

Child of Mine: Feeding with Love and Good Sense by Ellyn Satter (Boulder, CO: Bull Publishing Company, 2000).

Secrets of Feeding a Healthy Family: How to Eat, How to Raise Good Eaters, How to Cook by Ellyn Satter (Sun Prairie, WI: Kelcy Press, 2008).

Food Fights: Winning the Nutritional Challenges of Parenthood Armed with Insight, Humor, and a Bottle of Ketchup by Laura A. Jana, MD, FAAP, and Jennifer Shu, MD, FAAP (Itasca, IL: American Academy of Pediatrics, 2013).

Getting to YUM: The 7 Secrets of Raising Eager Eaters by Karen Le Billon (New York: William Morrow, 2014).

Hungry Monkey: A Food-Loving Father's Quest to Raise an Adventurous Eater by Matthew Amster-Burton (New York: Houghton Mifflin Harcourt, 2009).

Salt Sugar Fat: How the Food Giants Hooked Us by Michael Moss (New York: Random House, 2014).

Baby-Led Weaning: The Essential Guide to Introducing Solid Foods and Helping Your Baby to Grow Up a Happy and Confident Eater by Gill Rapley and Tracey Murkett (New York: The Experiment, 2010).

Fearless Feeding: How to Raise Healthy Eaters from High Chair to High School by Jill Castle and Maryann Jacobsen, MS, RD (San Francisco, CA: Jossey-Bass, 2013).

Happy Mealtimes with Happy Kids: How to Teach Your Child about the Joy of Food! by Melanie Potock, MA, CCC-SLP (My Munch Bug Publishing, 2014).

Food Chaining: The Proven 6-Step Plan to Stop Picky Eating, Solve Feeding Problems, and Expand Your Child's Diet by Cheryl Fraker, CCC-SLP, CLC, Mark Fishbein, MD, Sibyl Cox, RD, LD, CLC, and Laura Walbert, CCC-SLP, CLC (New York: Da Capo Lifelong, 2007).

Just Take a Bite: Easy, Effective Answers to Food Aversions and Eating Challenges! by Lori Ernsperger, PhD, and Tania Stegen-Hanson, OTR/L (Arlington, TX: Future Horizons, 2004).

Cookbooks for Kids

The Forest Feast for Kids: Colorful Vegetarian Recipes That Are Simple to Make by Erin Gleeson (New York: Abrams Books for Young Readers, 2016).

The Cultured Chef: An International Cookbook for Kids by Nicholas Beatty and Coleen McIntyre (Vancouver, WA: BookSprocket, 2014).

Salad People and More Real Recipes: A Cookbook for Preschoolers and Up by Mollie Katzen (Berkeley, CA, and Toronto: Tricycle Press, 2005).

Fanny at Chez Panisse: A Child's Restaurant Adventures with 46 Recipes by Alice Waters with Bob Carrau and Patricia Curtan (New York: HarperCollins, 1992).

Cooking with Curious Chef: Get Kids Really Cooking with Step by Step Recipes and Activities by Barbara J. Brandt, MEd (Hartland, WI: Tailor Made Products, Inc., 2016).

Cooking Class: 57 Fun Recipes Kids Will Love to Make (and Eat!) by Deanna F. Cook (North Adams, MA: Storey Publishing, 2015).

Let's Cook French: A Family Cookbook by Claudine Pépin (Beverly, MA: Quarry Books, 2016).

The Young Chef: Recipes and Techniques for Kids Who Love to Cook by the Culinary Institute of America and Mark Ainsworth (New York: Houghton Mifflin Harcourt, 2016).

Eat Your Greens, Reds, Yellows, and Purples: More Than 20 Vegetarian Recipes (London: DK Children, 2016).

Pretend Soup and Other Real Recipes: A Cookbook for Preschoolers and Up by Mollie Katzen and Ann Henderson (Berkeley, CA, and Toronto: Tricycle Press, 1994).

Alice Waters and the Trip to Delicious by Jacqueline Briggs Martin (Bellevue, WA: Readers to Eaters, 2014).

Cookbooks for Parents

The Waldorf School Book of Soups by Marsha Post and Andrea Huff (Great Barrington, MA: Bell Pond Books, 2006).

The Waldorf Book of Breads by Marsha Post and Winslow Eliot (Great Barrington, MA: SteinerBooks, 2009).

The Waldorf Cookbook by Kelly Sundstrom (CreateSpace Independent Publishing, 2009).

Plant-Powered Families: Over 100 Kid-Tested, Whole-Foods Vegan Recipes by Dreena Burton (Dallas, TX: BenBella Books, 2015).

The Pollan Family Table: The Best Recipes and Kitchen Wisdom for Delicious, Healthy Family Meals by Corky, Lori, Dana, and Tracy Pollan (New York: Scribner, 2014).

Weelicious: 140 Fast, Fresh, and Easy Recipes by Catherine McCord (New York: William Morrow, 2012).

What Chefs Feed Their Kids: Recipes and Techniques for Cultivating a Love of Good Food by Fanae Aaron (Guilford, CT: Lyons Press, 2012).

The Best Homemade Kids' Lunches on the Planet: Make Lunches Your Kids Will Love with More Than 200 Deliciously Nutritious Meal Ideas by Laura Fuentes (Beverly, MA: Fair Winds Press, 2014).

Little Foodie: Recipes for Babies and Toddlers with Taste by Michele Olivier with Sara Peternell, MNT (Berkeley, CA: Sonoma Press, 2015).

A Few More Cookbooks We Like

Home Made Summer by Yvette van Boven (New York: Stewart, Tabori & Chang, 2012).

Bountiful: Recipes Inspired by Our Garden by Todd Porter and Diane Cu (New York: Stewart, Tabori & Chang, 2013).

Salad for Dinner: Complete Meals for All Seasons by Jeanne Kelly (New York: Rizzoli International Publications, 2012).

Saladish: A Crunchier, Grainier, Herbier, Heartier, Tastier Way with Vegetables by Ilene Rosen with Donna Gelb (New York: Artisan, 2018).

Hipcooks: Around the World in 12 Dinner Parties by Monika Reti (Los Angeles: Hipcooks, 2012).

Six Seasons: A New Way with Vegetables by Joshua McFadden with Martha Holmberg (New York: Artisan, 2017).

The Pretty Dish: More Than 150 Everyday Recipes & 50 Beauty DIYs to Nourish Your Body Inside & Out by Jessica Merchant (New York: Rodale, 2018).

Half Baked Harvest Cookbook: Recipes from My Barn in the Mountains by Tieghan Gerard (New York: Clarkson Potter, 2017).

Children's Books Related to Food

Broc and Cara's Picnic Party by Dave A. Wilson (Dave Wilson Publishing, 2014).

Eating the Alphabet: Fruits & Vegetables from A to Z by Lois Ehlert (New York: HMH Books for Young Readers, 1993).

Pete the Cat: Pete's Big Lunch by James Dean (New York: HarperCollins, 2013).

The Gardener by Sarah Stewart (New York: Square Fish, 1997).

Wolfie's Secret by Nicola Senior (London: Faber & Faber, 2017).

Monsters Don't Eat Broccoli by Barbara Jean Hicks (New York: Dragonfly Books, 2009).

Jamberry by Bruce Degen (New York: HarperCollins, 1983).

Curious George and the Pizza Party by Margret and H.A. Rey and Cynthia Platt (New York: Houghton Mifflin Harcourt, 2010).

Spork by Kyo Maclear (Toronto: Kids Can Press, 2010).

The Carrot Seed by Ruth Krauss (New York: Harper & Row, 1945).

Stone Soup by Marcia Brown (New York: Aladdin Paperbacks, 1947).

Jojo and the Food Fight by Didier Lévy (Cambridge, MA: Barefoot Books, 2015).

There Are No Bears in This Bakery by Julia Sarcone-Roach (New York: Alfred A. Knopf, 2019).

Curious George Makes Pancakes by Margret and H. A. Rey (New York: Houghton Mifflin Harcourt, 1998).

Bread and Jam for Frances by Russell Hoban (New York: Harper & Row, 1964).

Cloudy with a Chance of Meatballs by Judi Barrett (New York: Atheneum Books for Young Readers, 1978).

The Bear Ate Your Sandwich by Julia Sarcone-Roach (New York: Alfred A. Knopf, 2015).

Little Chef by Matt Stine and Elisabeth Weinberg (New York: Feiwel and Friends, 2018).

Amelia Bedelia's First Apple Pie by Herman Parish (New York: Greenwillow Books, 2010).

Blueberries for Sal by Robert McCloskey (New York: Viking Press, 1948).

Thank You, Omu! by Oge Mora (New York: Little, Brown, 2018).

Chef Roy Choi and the Street Food Remix by Jacqueline Briggs Martin and June Jo Lee (Bellevue, WA: Readers to Eaters, 2017).

The Very Hungry Caterpillar by Eric Carle (New York: Philomel Books, 1969).

When Grandma Gives You a Lemon Tree by Jamie L. B. Deenihan (New York: Sterling Children's Books, 2019).

Bread Lab! by Kim Binczewski and Bethany Econopouly (Bellevue, WA: Readers to Eaters, 2018).

The Taco Stand by Tim S. Vasquez (Chandler, AZ: Toodaloo Publishing, 2019).

But I Don't Eat Ants by Dan Marvin (Brooklyn, NY: POW!, 2017).

In Our Mothers' House by Patricia Polacco (New York: Philomel Books, 2009).

Seven Silly Eaters by Mary Ann Hoberman (New York: HMH Books, 2000).

KITCHEN TOOLS
AND UTENSILS FOR KIDS

Montessori Services

This company has lots of high-quality wood and stainless kids' kitchen supplies, including our favorite kids' knife, a glass citrus juicer, and other prep items we love: www.montessoriservices .com/practical-life/food-preparation

For Small Hands

This company also has a good supply of kids' food-prep supplies and kid serving plates: www .forsmallhands.com/cooking/preparing-food

Opinel

Fancy knives for kids, including some wooden knives with finger guards: https://www.opinel -usa.com/collections/opinel-kids-corner

RESOURCES FOR KIDS WHO HAVE FEEDING CHALLENGES

Many food-related issues with children can be resolved when parents change the way they structure mealtime, menus, and set limits (see Chapter 2). However, if you feel you've tried everything and mealtime with your kids is still super stressful, don't despair.

If your kid eats less than twenty foods, avoids foods of a certain texture, gags when trying certain foods, cries at meals, has poor weight gain, or if there are frequent family fights about food, consider calling in a professional to help.

Sensory processing disorder is cited as one of the most common causes of extreme picky eating among kids. A balanced sensory system is key for learning to eat new foods, so if a child has some sensory processing issues, the sensations (sight, smell, taste, and texture) of food might be extra intense. Some professional resources that could help:

Find a speech-language pathologist or occupational therapist who specializes in feeding (may be classified as dysphagia): www.asha.org/findpro

Find a registered dietitian nutritionist: www.eatright.org/find-an-expert

Find an SOS (sequential oral sensory) therapist: sosapproach-conferences.com/parentscaregivers/therapist-referrals

Melanie Potock, My Munch Bug: mymunchbug.com

Marsha Dunn Klein, Mealtime Notions: www.mealtimenotions.com

The Ellyn Satter Institute: www.ellynsatterinstitute.org

Pediatrician Nimali Fernando (aka Doctor Yum): www.doctoryum.org

TIPS FOR MEALS WITH TODDLERS

Good luck getting your toddler to sit down for a civilized meal. Toddlers can be so busy and distractible that they really don't have any interest in sitting down to a meal. Most will tap out after five or ten minutes at the table, so you need to act fast!

Experts suggest:

Manage transitions. Let your toddler know that it'll be dinnertime in, say, fifteen minutes. Give a five-minute warning. Then say, "You can play later; now it's dinnertime."

If your toddler is having a tough time coming to the table, invite whatever toy he can't seem to leave behind—the train or the dinosaur—to come eat dinner, too.

Serve your toddler's food, then focus on enjoying your own meal and talking about other topics.

Toddlers will leave the table repeatedly if allowed. If this becomes a trend, allow one bathroom trip during dinner, but after that, if the kid leaves, say, "You left the table, showing us that you're done eating. We'll have a snack in a few hours." Hold firm.

If your toddler still doesn't want to come to the table, let her know that she doesn't have to eat but that you'd like her to keep you company for a few minutes while you eat. Set a timer, then let her go free after a few minutes if she still wants to.

Young toddlers might push their plates away, which usually means they're done eating. Older toddlers (two years plus) might want to be done but still be hungry. In that case, it's okay to encourage them to sit at the table a bit longer without forcing them or pressuring them to eat anything.

Let your toddler choose how much and what to eat—as long as it's chosen from what you've served him.

Let toddlers eat their own way—they'll likely use their hands and make a mess.

Ideally, by the time a kid leaves toddlerhood, he or she will have developed a few food-related competencies: a positive attitude about eating, a reliance on internal hunger and fullness to know how much to eat, a reliance on variations in appetite to know what to eat, the ability to enjoy many different foods, the ability to try new foods and learn to like them, and the ability to "make do" with less than favorite foods.

FOOD FIELD TRIPS

Take your family on a food-related field trip. A few ideas to get you started:

Harley Farms Goat Dairy—Pescadero, CA

The farm offers a tour of the edible garden, barn, goats, and milking parlor.

http://www.harleyfarms.com

Ben & Jerry's—Waterbury, VT

This ice cream company offers a factory tour that's open to the public.

https://www.benjerry.com/about-us/factory-tours

Pez Visitor Center—Orange, CT

This candy manufacturer is home to the largest PEZ memorabilia on public display in the world, the world's largest PEZ candy dispenser, and a viewing area for seeing into the candy production area.

https://us.pez.com/pages/hours-and-location

Jelly Belly Factory—Fairfield, CA

This jelly bean company offers free tours of the factory.

jellybelly.com/californiafactory

Julius Strugis Pretzel Bakery—Lititz, PA

This company offers free pretzel tours that include a pretzel-twisting lesson.

https://juliussturgis.com/plan-your-visit

Bob's Red Mill—Milwaukie, OR

This flour company offers kids a chance to see a flour mill in action and to learn about stone-milling and whole grains.

bobsredmill.com

Creo Chocolate—Portland, OR

This chocolate factory offers an interactive tour of how chocolate is made from freshly roasted cacao beans.

https://creochocolate.com

Tillamook Cheese Factory—Tillamook, OR

This cheese company offers tours of its factory and a chance to see forty-pound blocks of cheese move through the production process.

https://www.tillamook.com

Intelligentsia Coffee—Chicago, IL

This coffee company offers a live demonstration of the roasting process.

https://www.intelligentsiacoffee.com/chicago -roasting-works-tour

Shatto Milk Company—Osborn, MO

This milk company offers a tour of the processing plant, which shows how bottles are prepped and how cows are milked. Meet some cows in the process.

https://shattomilk.com/events-tours

Albanese Candy Factory— Merrillville, IN

This candy company offers a public tour of gummi manufacturing.

https://www.albanesecandy.com/factory-tours

Two Hives Honey—Austin, TX

This honey company teaches families about honey bees and includes hands-on exploration of an active beehive.

https://www.twohiveshoney.com/hive-tours

Temecula Olive Oil Company— Aguanga, CA

This olive oil company offers guided walks through its olive groves along with lessons about olive harvesting techniques, milling, and pressing.

https://www.temeculaoliveoil.com/book-a-tour

Homeboy Industries— Los Angeles, CA

This company works with high-risk adults, who were once involved in gangs, and offers a tour that includes their bakery.

homeboyindustries.org

E. Waldo Ward & Son— Sierra Madre, CA

This jam and jelly company offers families a tour that shows how jams and jellies are made.

https://www.waldoward.com/ContactUs.aspx

Fallen Fruit—Los Angeles, CA

Fallen Fruit is an art collective that maps "public fruit" hanging over public walkways. Download a map and spend the day foraging fruit with your family.

www.fallenfruit.org

UNIVERSAL CONVERSION CHART

Oven Temperature Equivalents

250°F = 120°C   325°F = 160°C   400°F = 200°C   475°F = 240°C

275°F = 135°C   350°F = 180°C   425°F = 220°C   500°F = 260°C

300°F = 150°C   375°F = 190°C   450°F = 230°C

Measurement Equivalents

Measurements should always be level unless directed otherwise.

⅛ teaspoon = 0.5 mL

¼ teaspoon = 1 mL

½ teaspoon = 2 mL

1 teaspoon = 5 mL

1 tablespoon = 3 teaspoons = ½ fluid ounce = 15 mL

2 tablespoons = ⅛ cup = 1 fluid ounce = 30 mL

4 tablespoons = ¼ cup = 2 fluid ounces = 60 mL

5⅓ tablespoons = ⅓ cup = 3 fluid ounces = 80 mL

8 tablespoons = ½ cup = 4 fluid ounces = 120 mL

10⅔ tablespoons = ⅔ cup = 5 fluid ounces = 160 mL

12 tablespoons = ¾ cup = 6 fluid ounces = 180 mL

16 tablespoons = 1 cup = 8 fluid ounces = 240 mL

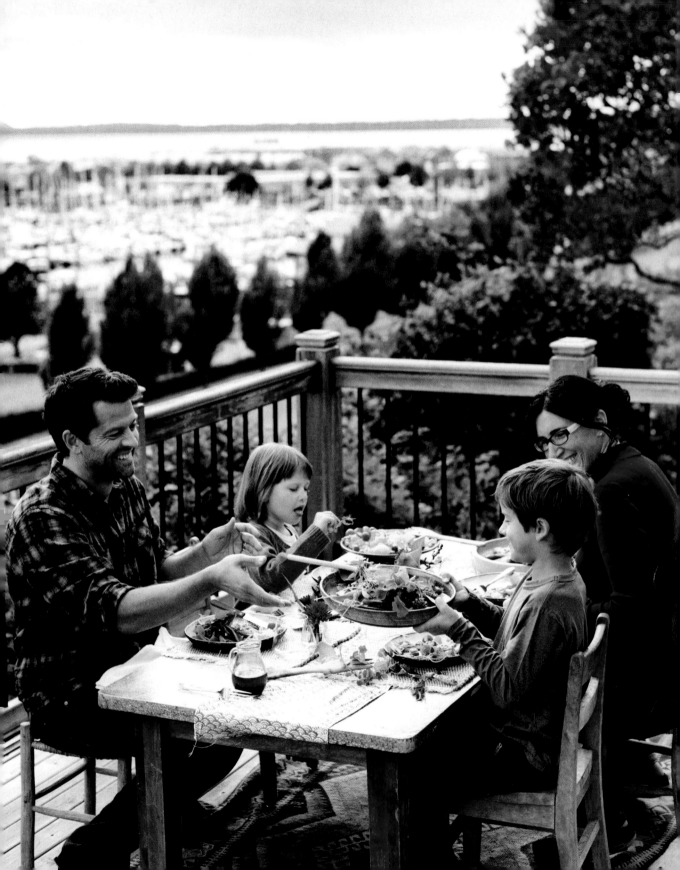

ACKNOWLEDGMENTS

We couldn't have written this book without a gaggle of food-loving, open-minded friends and collaborators. Thank you, Kathryn, for essentially daring us to write this. We're grateful to photographer Michèle M. Waite, who goes by Misha (yes, this project involved two Mishas), for her devotion to good food, humor, and natural sunlight. Misha, you are a true wonder of the Pacific Northwest. We're thankful for our longtime friend Marne Dupere, who tirelessly insists on beauty even when everything is being pelted by rain. Julie H. and team: thank you all for your attention to detail, and for your joyful, collaborative spirits. Special thanks to consulting chef Ryan Ross for her enthusiasm and passion for this project. We're grateful to Darius, dad friend/former chef, who stayed up into the wee hours talking about how to cook real food for children. Catalina and Luz: thank you for sharing your enthusiasm about food with our family.

Jean G.: thanks for being a seasoned culinary resource, and for refining recipes with us. Thanks to Kristina Meltzer, stylish mother of three, for making our kids look less disheveled. Thanks to Byrd Leavell and Jacob Fenton at UTA for helping us find a home for this book. To our editors Libby Edelson and Sydney Rogers: thank you for ushering this book from idea to completion and for such thoughtful feedback along the way. Thanks to everyone at HC for making this book beautiful and for helping us put it out into the world. (We should note that any mistakes in this book are all their fault.)

We appreciate Misha's mom for her determination to make food with love—even when she was homeless with two young children and food seemed impossible. We're indebted to our offspring, West and Maison, not only for inspiring us to embrace wild, adventurous cooking, but for making us laugh every single day. We're especially grateful to all the children in our little Pacific Northwest hamlet for bravely tasting new recipes with us. (Eternal thanks to our eleven-year-old neighbor, Ella: if you hadn't told us that beet popsicle tasted like dirt, it'd still be included in this cookbook. Aspiring chefs everywhere thank you!) We feel lucky to be surrounded by so many families who are game to partake in our hair-brained food shenanigans. Thank you for loaning us a friendly, photogenic chicken; for sharing your secrets to irresistible broccoli; for introducing us to culinary novelties like geoduck sushi and deep-fried caviar; for serving your kids fried eggs on pizza without flinching; and for reminding us to bring the spirit of adventure to family life . . . and to food.

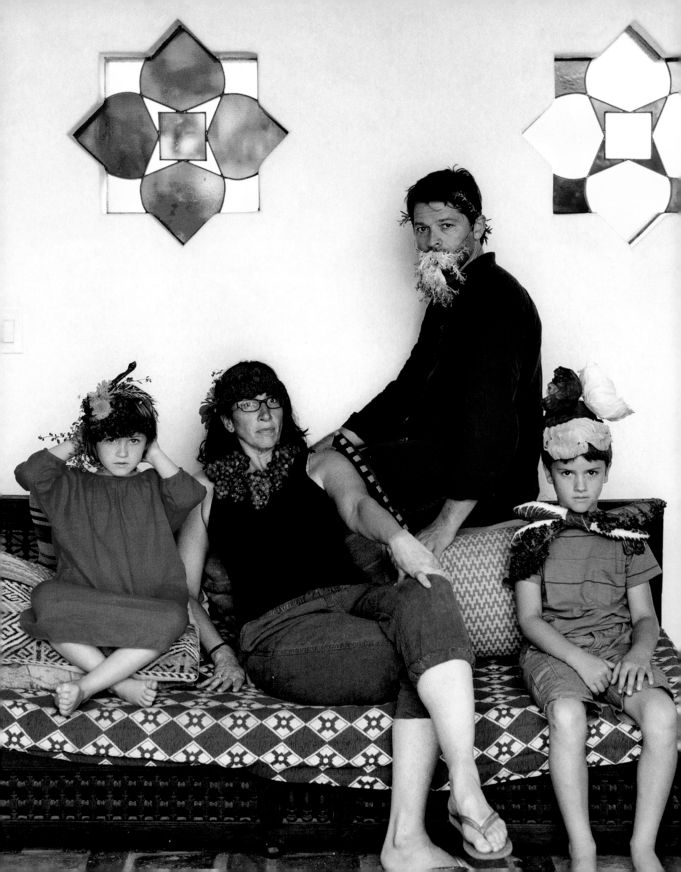

ABOUT THE
AUTHORS AND CHEFS

*M*isha Collins first made a name for himself as an actor on the hit TV show *Supernatural*. Known for his irreverent humor, Misha has become a personality on social media and relishes inspiring people to take on absurd, challenging, and generally inadvisable tasks. Misha is also known for Random Acts (RA), the nonprofit organization he founded, which aims to inspire random acts of kindness big and small. RA has built an orphanage in Haiti and a school in Nicaragua, and continues to tackle larger projects around the world. In addition, Misha founded the Greatest International Scavenger Hunt the World Has Ever Seen (GISHWHES), an annual scavenger hunt that has drawn hundreds of thousands of participants from more than one hundred countries. GISHWHES has won seven Guinness World Records, including the largest online scavenger hunt ever and the longest chain of paper clips ever. He's also been known to trap his family and friends in the kitchen for twelve-hour jam-making sessions when blackberries are in season.

Vicki Collins, Misha's coconspirator and mom of West and Maison, has a background in history and journalism. She's written about everything from fingernail fashion to architectural history for publications such as *The Washington Post*, *U.S. News & World Report*, and the *Los Angeles Times*. She holds a PhD in US history. She came to the kitchen late in life, but with the help of two young avant-garde chefs, she's come to enjoy cooking family meals.

West Collins (age eight) has been cooking since he was two years old. West's cooking antics can be seen in several episodes of the Web series *Cooking Fast & Fresh with West*. When a toddler is given carte blanche in the kitchen, meals become . . . innovative and often inedible. West likes audiobooks, Legos, and salad.

Maison Collins (age six) is a budding chef in her own right—she chimes in as critic in this book and has developed her own not at all critically acclaimed recipes such as parsley-beet-cinnamon muffins. She says she likes cooking so much she might work in a restaurant someday—if she doesn't follow through on her other passion, tracking bats.